Chinese Traditional Healing – Continued

# Sir Henry Wellcome Asian Series

The titles published in this series are listed at *brill.com/was*

# Chinese Traditional Healing – Continued

*A Survey of Manuscripts 8840 to 8960 of the*
*Staatsbibliothek zu Berlin*

*Edited by*

Paul U. Unschuld
Zheng Jinsheng

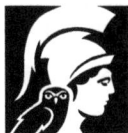

BRILL

LEIDEN | BOSTON

Cover illustration: Page of Ms. 8857. Yi xue yuan li, Medical principles, by Ming Wang Ji, 1601.

The Library of Congress Cataloging-in-Publication Data is available online at https://catalog.loc.gov
LC record available at https://lccn.loc.gov/2025020020

Typeface for the Latin, Greek, and Cyrillic scripts: "Brill". See and download: brill.com/brill-typeface.

ISSN 1570-1484
ISBN 978-90-04-73638-2 (paperback)
ISBN 978-90-04-73709-9 (e-book)
DOI 10.1163/9789004737099

# CONTENTS

# Preliminary Remarks

This survey offers detailed information on 121 volumes held by the Staatsbibliothek zu Berlin as part of the Berlin Collections of Manuscript Volumes from the 16th through the Early 20th Century. The volumes introduced here were prepared in the 19th and early 20th century. They cover a broad range of fields in traditional Chinese health care, including a large number of apotropaic contents.

In 2012, the publisher of this study, Brill, Leiden, published a three-volume catalog of the Berlin collections. It describes 881 volumes from the collection of the Staatsbibliothek zu Berlin and 58 volumes from the Ethnologisches Museum Berlin. The volumes described here bring the total number of volumes described in detail to 1062. I later donated a final part of the collection to the Staatsbibliothek; a detailed description of these more than 100 volumes is still pending. All volumes are available in the central catalog of the Staatsbibliothek under the search term "Sammlung Unschuld". They are being successively digitized and can therefore be viewed worldwide.

Interest in this unique collection is constantly growing. In fact, these handwritten records of healers, apothecaries, private individuals and other groups represent a very valuable collection. They are texts that can be regarded as extremely meaningful documents of the real practice of medicine in China in the last centuries before the founding of the People's Republic of China.

All these records were written by hand because the authors considered them worthy of further attention. Medical prescriptions, acupuncture and tuina therapies as well as apotropaic spells and various techniques that were believed to be able to influence one's own body or that of others in the desired way are collected here because the healers, apothecaries and laymen were convinced of their effectiveness. This is of particular interest today, as there are tens of thousands of healing recipes containing mainly herbal ingredients. Over the centuries, experience with effects on the human organism has accumulated here, which can now be verified and evaluated using modern scientific methods.

Based on these handwritten records, an interdisciplinary team of developers, statisticians, and experts in theory and history of Chinese medicine of the Institute of Chinese Life Sciences at Charité-Universitätsmedizin Berlin has entered over 41,000 formulae with around 3,700 substance names and over 12,000 synonyms of dialectal origin into a database. The data input was realized through a custom designed semi-automated procedure, carefully combining text-mining methods with indispensable expert interpretation due to the forgotten regional naming of substances and disease names. By organizing the historical material in such a categorical and relational manner, findings on statistical causal relationships and thus on the mode of action of individual substances as well as on synergistic effects of combinations of several substances in individual formulae can be obtained with the help of state-of-the-art data-mining algorithms and established methods from network science. Since 2015, the Institute, together with several scientific and industrial partners, has posed questions to this database and received answers that are of great interest to pharmacology and industrial application, including a patent and leads on plants not known anymore in modern TCM that are considered for drug development. The Institute is open to corresponding collaborations and contract research.

The value of the collection for research into the history of medical therapies in China cannot be overestimated. Each individual manuscript bears witness to the reception of historical therapeutic knowledge and ideas by individual healers and patients. These documentations have a different significance than the many printed books in which medical theory and practice were disseminated.

The manuscripts reveal the extent to which daily use implemented the knowledge of the books or took other paths. The Berlin collection contains numerous copies of older printed works, sometimes written down many centuries after their last documented printing. Often there are personal annotations by the people who produced the manuscript, or they are excerpts with omissions that are also significant. The fact that the manuscripts express a social reality that is hardly recognizable in the printed literature is also demonstrated by the many prescriptions for premature abortion, which were apparently in great demand and used on a large scale.

The structure of the individual entries in the overview presented here follows the pattern of the 2012 publication, providing information on the title of a manuscript, its ID in the Staatsbibliothek, the type of subject it deals with, the appearance and type of binding, the measurements, the presence of a title page and the number of pages, the number of lines per page and the number of characters per line, the author and date, as well as an overview of the contents and concluding remarks on the age of the volume.

In contrast to the 2012 publication, each individual manuscript description is accompanied

By one or more illustrations that provide an indication of the quality of the calligraphy and drawings in the text. We are convinced that this will make it much easier to assess each individual manuscript and its potential suitability for more detailed analysis. Two appendices make it easy to search for titles and names of individuals. An additional appendix with key terms helps in the search for topics documented in the manuscripts that may be of interest to researchers and other readers.

As in 2012, I would like to point out at this point that this continuation of the individual descriptions of the manuscripts was only possible as a joint effort in collaboration with my esteemed colleague Prof. Zheng Jinsheng. Only Prof. Zheng Jinsheng was able to read the individual manuscripts and evaluate them in response to our questions. I was left with the task of translating his notes, asking further questions and preparing all the material fo publication in the way we have now presented it.

We are indebted to the German Research Association (DFG) for funding the project (UN 33/32-1) leading to this result.

The text for this volume was completed in 2015. Then, for almost ten years, my attention was focused exclusively on the translation of the *Ben cao gang mu* 本草纲目. We are indebted to Brill and anonymous reviewers for the publication of this volume.


Berlin, November 2024
Paul U. Unschuld

## Abbreviations

ID:                    Idenfication Number, Staatsbibliothek zu Berlin

L.P./CH.L:             Lines per page/characters per line


Note: Titles of manuscript volumes given in brackets ( .... ) were tentatively assigned to volumes without explicit titles stated on their covers

# A Survey of Manuscripts #8840 to #8960

| | |
|---|---|
| TITLE: | *Dou tai shi chuang yang jing yan quan shu* 竇太師瘡瘍經驗全書， The Grand Teacher Dou's proven complete writings on lesions and ulcers. |
| ID: | 8840 |
| CONTENTS: | External Medicine |
| APPEARANCE: | Ancient manuscript volume. Contents identical with ms. 8854. Identification of chapter missing. Margins torn; front page dilapidated. Average handwriting. |
| BINDING: | Thread |
| MEASURE: | 22.5 x. 13.0 |
| TITLE PAGE: | Blank |
| NO. OF PAGES: | 47 |
| L.P. /CH.L: | 7 x approx. 32 |
| LAYOUT: | No lines, no frames |

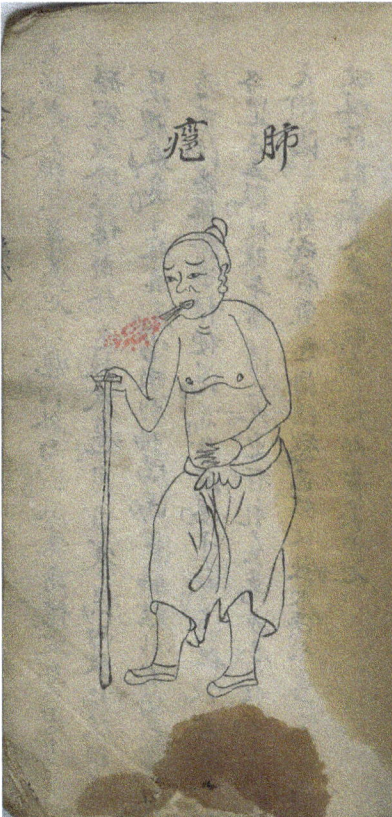

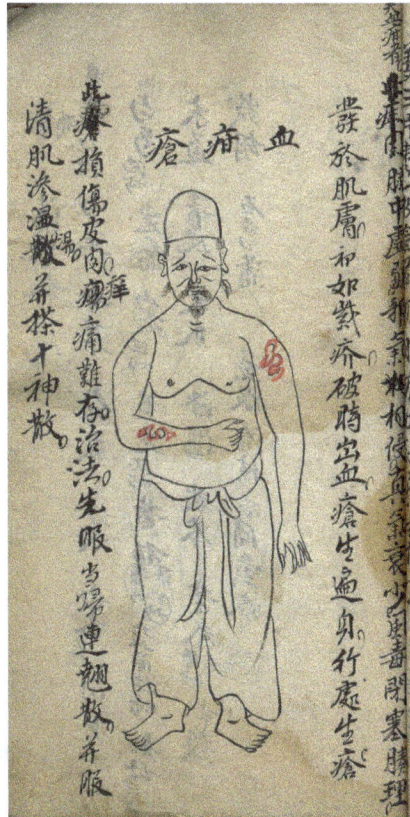

© PAUL U. UNSCHULD AND ZHENG JINSHENG, 2025 | DOI:10.1163/9789004737099_002

AUTHOR AND YEAR OF TEXT:

Ming, Dou Menglin 竇夢麟 with later addenda.

YEAR OF COPY:    Identical with Ms. 8854. Republican period.

SURVEY OF CONTENTS: A comparison shows that this is the 3rd *juan* of *Dou tai shi chuang yang jing yan quan shu* 竇太師瘡瘍經驗全書. It begins with the paragraph on *fei ju* 肺疽, "lung impediment-illness", and ends with *bi mian du* 鼻面毒, "nose and face poisoning". It informs of a total of 42 types of lesions. Numerous full-body drawings show the location, often marked with red dots, of a lesion, with lengthy explanations on their nature and pharmaceutical treatment. Additional comments to the drawings are meant to clarify further issues. For example, the illustration of *wei yong* 胃癰, "stomach obstruction-illness" is explained as *ci bing zai nei* 此病在內, "This disease is in the interior." Such information is quite noteworthy. The term 癰 *yong* has been translated as "welling abscess" in many English writings on historical Chinese medicine. The fact is, an "abscess" may be the result of an "obstruction-illness" because where the flow of qi is obstructed the blocked qi may accumulate and eventually break out as an abscess. However, the underlying problem is an "obstruction-illness" that may be situated somewhere deep in the human body.

***

TITLE:             *Tai yi shen zhen fang* 太乙神鍼方, Recipes for Taiyi's Divine Needle.

ID:                8841

CONTENTS:          Acupuncture

APPEARANCE:        Ancient manuscript. Crude hand-made paper. Cover dilapidated. Average handwriting.

BINDING:           Thread

MEASURE:           24.0 x. 13.0

TITLE PAGE:        Blank

NO. OF PAGES:      6

L.P. /CH.L:        8 x approx. 19

LAYOUT:            No lines, no frames

AUTHOR AND YEAR OF TEXT:

Qing, Fan Yuqi 范毓馪 (Peilan 培兰)

YEAR OF COPY:    See above.

SURVEY OF CONTENTS: This ms. has four prefaces and postscripts. They enable one to trace its history and contents. The first preface was written by Zhou Yonghe 周雍和 of Eastern Zhejiang for "the *Tai yi shen zhen* 太乙神針 compiled by the honorable [Mr.] Fan 范". A second preface was written by Qiu Shimin 邱時敏 of Huaiyang 淮陽 in the year *xinhai* 辛亥 of the *qianlong* 乾隆 reign period (1791). He had obtained the text and had ordered it to be printed. At the end of the text a man named Ai Xianfu 哀賢甫 is identified (according to bibliographical reference works this should be Ai Zhifu 袁質甫) as editor. Finally, there are two postscripts by Ye Gui 葉圭 from Cangzhou 滄州, dated 6th year of *xianfeng* 咸豐 reign period (1856), and by Sun Fuqing 孫福清 dated 2nd year of *tongzhi* 同治 reign period (1863). Hence this is the *Tai yi shen zhen fang* 太乙神針方 by the Qing author Fan Yuqi 范毓犄, listed in the *Zhong guo zhong yi gu ji zong mu* 中國中醫古籍總目.

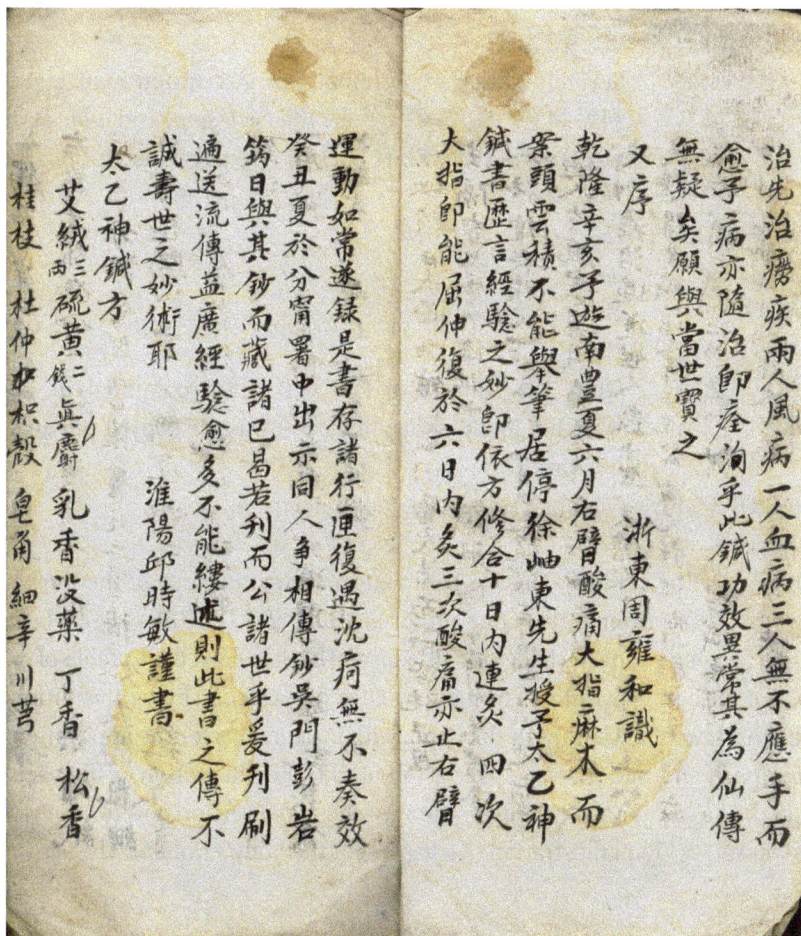

The so-called "Taiyi's divine needle", *Tai yi shen zhen* 太乙神針, is a cylindrical roll used in moxibustion therapy since the Ming dynasty. Its use spread rapidly in subsequent centuries. The contents of the present manuscript attest to the popularity of this new mode of the application of moxa-cauterization.

***

TITLE:            *You ke tie jing* 幼科鐵鏡, Iron mirror of pediatrics.
ID:               8842
CONTENTS:         Pediatrics
APPEARANCE:       Ancient manuscript. Pocket size. Aged paper color. Average handwriting.
BINDING:          Thread
MEASURE:          13 x 9.2
TITLE PAGE:       Severely damaged. Remnants of inscription readable: "幼科鐵鏡卷之二/禹鑄氏手書, *You ke tie jing*, 2nd *juan*. Handwritten by Mr. Yu Zhu." Back of title page: inscription: 阮茂遠佩/張子房
NO. OF PAGES:     124
L.P. /CH.L:       8 x 18
LAYOUT:           No lines, no frames
AUTHOR AND YEAR OF TEXT:
                  Qing, Xia Ding 夏鼎 (Yu Zhu 禹鑄) compiled in 1695. Whether Ruan Maoyuan 阮茂遠 was the copyist remains to be examined.
YEAR OF COPY:     No taboos observed. Republican era.

SURVEY OF CONTENTS: This is a complete, handwritten copy of the *You ke tie jing* 幼科鐵鏡 written by the Qing author Xia Ding 夏鼎 (Yu Zhu 禹鑄). It begins with a facsimile copy of the book's title page. This is followed by a table of contents of the book's five *juan*. The main text itself is preceded by an illustration of a face and two illustrations of the palm, with instructions for the application of *tuina*-push-and-pull massage. This is followed by an illustration of the back of a hand, of a lower arm with illustrations of the two insertion points *he gu* 合谷 and *hu kou* 虎口, an illustration of a leg and of the body's front and back.

The main text of *juan* 1 begins with a paragraph on the prognosis of fatal conditions, secret instructions transmitted in the home of Zhuo Xi, a poem on how to replace the intake of pharmaceutical drugs by push-and-pull massage, and the further paragraphs of the original text. At the end of the five *juan* a numbered list of 75 pharmaceutical recipes is copied. The recipes offer only the name and the ingredients of the prescriptions. There is no information on amounts or application. The *You ke tie jing* 幼科鐵鏡 was widely distributed towards the end of the Qing dynasty. Hence it was copied in numerous hand-written versions.

*\*\**

| | |
|---|---|
| TITLE: | *Zu chuan* 祖傳, Transmitted by the ancestors. |
| ID: | 8843 (1-2) |
| CONTENTS: | External medicine, Pharmaceutical recipes |
| APPEARANCE: | 2 vols. Ancient manuscript with a recent thread binding retaining though the old cover. Cover of vol. 1 with faint inscription in black ink: 祖傳/民旺卅. Handwriting above average. No table of contents. Numerous personal seals have been printed on characters throughout the text. Identifiable seal inscriptions are 陳栖印 and 倪化章. That is, Chen Qi 陳栖 and Ni Hua 倪化 may have been former owners of these volumes. |
| BINDING: | Thread |
| MEASURE: | 20.7 x 11.0 |
| TITLE PAGE: | No |
| NO. OF PAGES: | Vol. 1: 40 pp.; vol. 2: 35 pp. |
| L.P. /CH.L: | 6 x approx. 19 |
| LAYOUT: | No lines, no frames |
| AUTHOR AND YEAR OF TEXT: | |
| | Unknown |
| YEAR OF COPY: | No Qing era taboos observed. Republican era. |

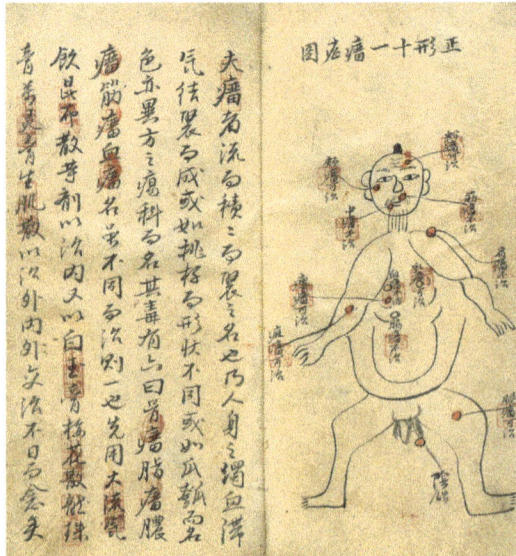

SURVEY OF CONTENTS: The structure of both volumes is identical. Page numbers have been added by a later person with blue fountain pen ink. First an illustration of a person shows the location and names of numerous illnesses. These conditions are then discussed in detail on the following pages. Vol. 1 has three such illustrations with subsequent explanations; vol. 2 has four such sections. The three sections of vol. 1 begin with an "illustration of ten pathological conditions with back view of a person," *fu xing shi zheng tu* 伏刑 (erroneous writing of: 形) 十症圖. Illness signs shown are 對口瘡、上搭手、下搭手、囊發, et al. Second illustration: 正面十二（症）圖. Illness signs shown are 眉發、胸發、乳發, et al. Third illustration: 正面十二症圖. Illness signs shown are 頂癧、螻蛄上串、螻蛄中串、螻蛄下串、痔漏, et al. In all, 80 illness signs are shown and discussed in terms of signs and pharmaceutical treatment. At the end of vol. 1 a note is added in small characters: "I cured a woman with sheep utter piles. All recipes employed failed to show an effect. Hence I conceptualized the following formula: *Dang gui*, 4 *liang*; *qin jiao*, 4 *liang*; *zhuang huang*, half raw, half processed, 3 *liang*; *huang qin* heated with wine, 3 *liang*. Dry all ingredients in the sun, and grind them together to a fine powder. Prepare pills with honey and have [the patient] ingest two pills with an empty stomach. After two dosages the cure was achieved." 予治一女人羊奶痔，諸方不效，想出此方：當歸四兩，秦艽四兩，莊黃半生熟三兩，黃芩酒炒三兩，曬燥共為細末，蜜丸空心服二單二癒. Apparently, the writer of these volumes was a practicing physician. The contents of vol. 2 begin with an "illustration of eleven pathological conditions with side view of a person," *ce xing shi yi zheng tu* 側形十一症圖. Illness signs shown are 眉風毒、耳門癰、中肩發、內臁瘡、外臁瘡, et al. Second "illustration of five pathological conditions with side view of a person," *ce xing wu zheng tu* 側形五症圖. Illness signs shown: 跳針毒、瘰癧、結喉癰、臀癰、指風刺. Third "illustration of seven pathological conditions with side view of a person," *ce xing qi zheng tu* 側形七症圖. Illness signs shown: 白面疔、馬刀、項癰, et al. Fourth "illustration of thirteen pathological conditions with front view of a person," *zheng xing shi san zheng tu* 正形十三症圖. Illness signs shown: 上眼丹、下眼丹、便毒、鬢發、乳癖, et al. In all, this volume comprises information on 50 pathological conditions and recipes.

The two volumes constitute the first half of a set of four volumes.

***

TITLE:           (see 8843, vols. 1 and 2)
ID:              8843 (3-4)
CONTENTS:        External medicine, Pharmaceutical recipes
APPEARANCE:      2 vols. Ancient manuscript with recent thread binding and new cover. No title. No table of contents. Handwriting above average. Numerous personal seals have been printed on characters throughout the text. Identifiable seal inscriptions are 陳栖印 and 倪化章. That is, Chen Qi 陳栖 and Ni Hua 倪化 may have been former owners of these volumes.
BINDING:         Thread
MEASURE:         20.5 x 10.9
TITLE PAGE:      No.
NO. OF PAGES:    Vol. 1: 38; vol. 2: 37
L.P. /CH.L:      6 x approx. 19
LAYOUT:          No lines, no frames
AUTHOR AND YEAR OF TEXT:
                 Unknown
YEAR OF COPY:    The absence of characters written to observe Qing dynasty taboos and other signs suggest that these volumes were written during the Republican era.

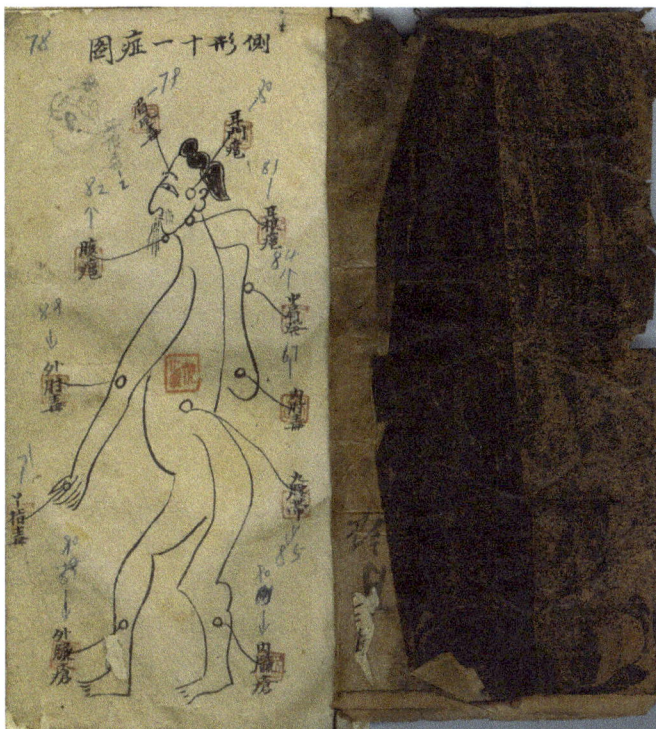

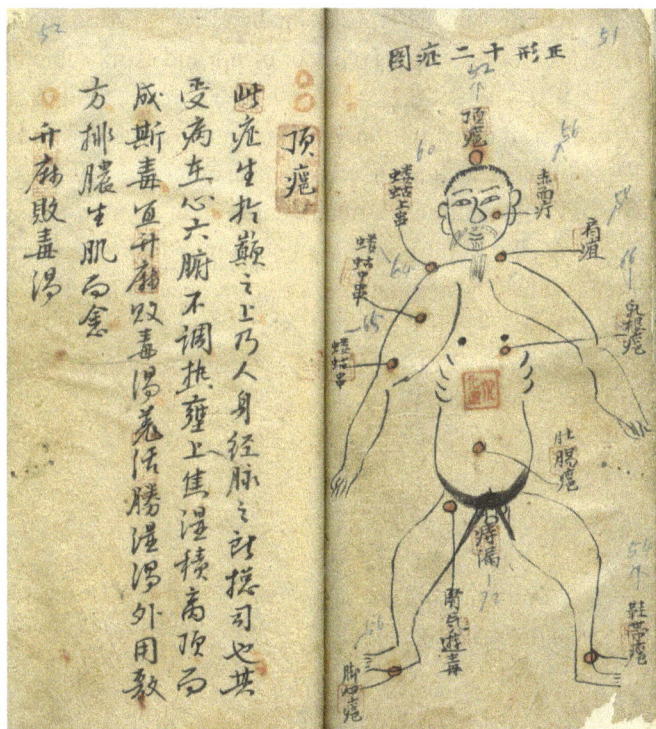

SURVEY OF CONTENTS: First and final pages missing. The structure shows that these two volumes belong with 8843 vol. 1 and 2 to a set of four volumes. The first conditions discussed, i.e., "knee and leg pain," *xi tui tong* 膝腿痛 and "ankle poison," *jiao huai du* 腳踝毒, are the final two mentioned in the "illustration of thirteen pathological conditions with front view of a person," *zheng xing shi yi zheng tu* 正形十三症圖 of vol. 2 of 8843. These are followed by an "illustration of eleven pathological conditions with front view of a person," *zheng xing shi yi zheng tu* 正形十一瘤症圖 with conditions shown and identified as "can be treated/cured", "cannot be treated/cured", such as 粉瘤可治、筋瘤不治、乳瘤可治、血瘤不治, etc. Subsequent illustrations are: the "illustration of three pathological conditions of females," *nü ren san zheng tu* 女人三症圖, with three conditions shown: 頭風、內吹、外吹，并出方劑. Second: "illustration of three pathological conditions of females," *nü ren san zheng tu* 女人三症圖, with three conditions shown: 鼠瘡、乳癰、陰蝕. Third: "illustration of seven pathological conditions with side view of a person," *ce xing qi zheng tu* 側形七症圖, with 7 conditions shown, plus pharmaceutical recipes. Fourth: "fourteen pathological conditions of children," *xiao er shi si zheng* 小兒十四症, with ten conditions shown.

These sections are followed by a section 楊梅瘡及諸般惡瘡等症秘方, "Secret recipes for syphilis and all types of malign sores", listing more than 90 pharmaceutical recipes for various types of ulcers and skin problems, such as 紫白癜風、白面雀斑、陰風、體氣、腸風下血、白禿瘡、梅花瘡、頭瘡, as well as those to be used for conditions encountered in gynecology and internal medicine. Some of these recipes are well known; others are folk prescriptions.

The fourth and final volume is a documentation of approximately 180 recipes, mostly for swelling and poisoning encountered in external medicine. However, there are further therapeutic indications such as 絞腸痧、牙疼、乳蛾、痢疾、癬、陰癢、黃泡瘡、痔漏、內吹、大麻風、喉痛、婦人茄病、肺癰、肺痿、天皰瘡、婦人白帶、人面瘡、胃氣痛, etc. from internal and external medicine.

\*\*\*

TITLE:     *Dou zhen jing yan liang fang* 痘疹經驗良方, Proven recipes for smallpox papules.

ID:     8844

CONTENTS:     Pox

APPEARANCE:     Ancient manuscript. The edges where the binding is are severely damaged. Cover with inscription: 痘疹經驗良方/天保堂. Main text: average handwriting but very careful.

BINDING:     Thread

MEASURE:     18.4 x 13.0

TITLE PAGE:     No.

NO. OF PAGES:     47

L.P. /CH.L:     8 x 16

LAYOUT:     No lines, no margins

AUTHOR AND YEAR OF TEXT:

The title of this volume is listed in the bibliography *Zhong guo zhong yi gu ji zong mu* 中國中醫古籍總目 only once as "(秘传)小儿痘疹经验良方", written by the Yuan era author Wei Junyong 魏君用. Only two copies are known to exist in Chinese libraries, one in 上海圖書館, the other in 中國中醫科學院圖書館.

YEAR OF COPY:     No Qing dynasty taboos observed. Republican era.

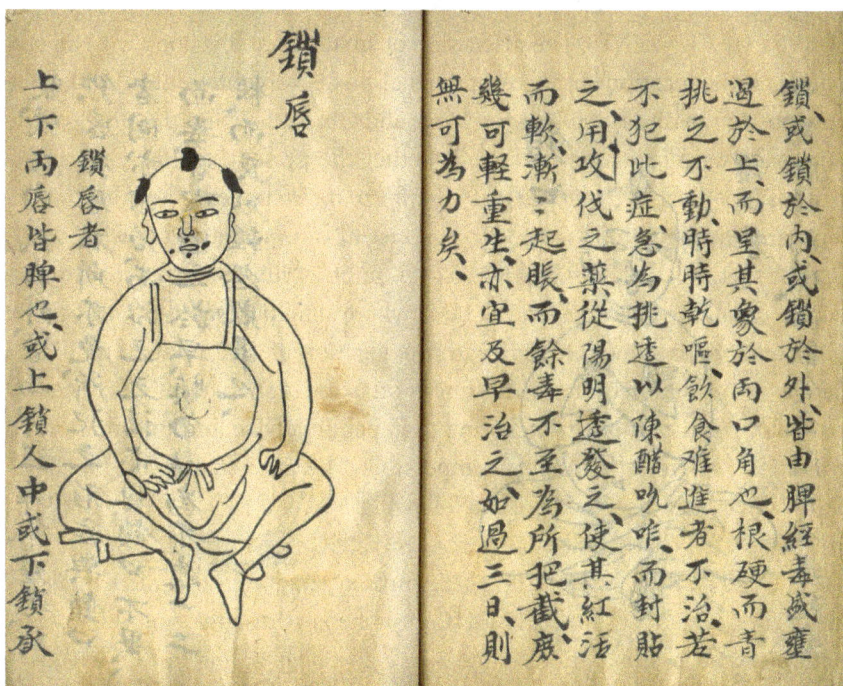

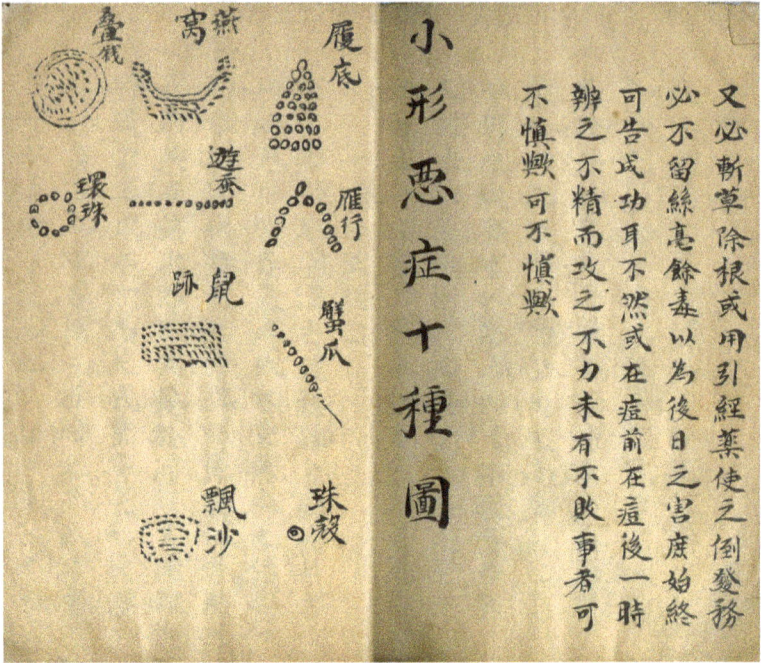

SURVEY OF CONTENTS: The discussion of smallpox in this book with an emphasis on the locations of the eruptions of pox is very different from the discussions of the disease during the Ming and Qing eras when the times of the outbreaks were of major concern. Whether the present volume is indeed a copy of Wei Junyong's original text remains to be examined. The table of contents and the main items treated in the present volume are as follows:

First section: 二十四圖總論. A discussion of 24 illustrations. This is a discourse on all the locations on the body where smallpox papules may appear. The illustrations show the body with the location of an eruption and offer a detailed explanation of the significance of that location in terms of theoretical physiology and pathology, including therapeutic advice and information on conditions where a treatment is impossible. The designations of the conditions shown and discussed are the following: 蒙頭, 覆釜, 抱鬢, 蒙【骨丸】, 托腮, 托頷, 鎖口, 鎖唇, 鎖項, 鎖咽, 披肩, 攢胸, 攢背, 囊腹, 纏腰, 囊毬, 鎖肛, 鱗坐, 抱膝, 抱脛, 兩截, 無跟, 四空, 四實. Further paragraphs include Er shi si tu zhi fa zong lun 二十四圖治法總論, "Comprehensive discourse on therapeutic patterns, with 24 illustrations", Xiao xing e zheng shi zhong tu 小形惡症十種圖, "Ten illustrations of small size malign disease conditions," and Shi tu zhi fa zong lun 十圖治法總論, "Comprehensive discourse on therapeutic patterns with 10 illustrations," followed by a listing of more than 20 recipes.

\*\*\*

| | |
|---|---|
| TITLE: | *Tie da sun shang. Xue dao shang* 跌打損傷·穴道傷, Injuries from falls and blows. Injuries received at the insertion holes and pathways. |
| ID: | 8845 |
| CONTENTS: | Bone setting; traumatology |
| APPEARANCE: | Ancient manuscript. Edges slightly damaged. Cover added by later person, with careless handwriting: 杂症良方, "Good recipes for diverse conditions". Main text: average handwriting. |
| BINDING: | Thread |
| MEASURE: | 23.5 x 12.1 |
| TITLE PAGE: | No |
| NO. OF PAGES: | 101 |
| L.P. /CH.L: | First half of volume: 9 x approx. 20. Latter part: various sections with larger and smaller characters. |
| LAYOUT: | No lines, no frames |
| AUTHOR AND YEAR OF TEXT: | |
| | Qing, Author: Shao Qinjun 邵勤俊. Copyist: unknown |
| YEAR OF COPY: | No Qing dynasty tabooos observed. Republican era. |

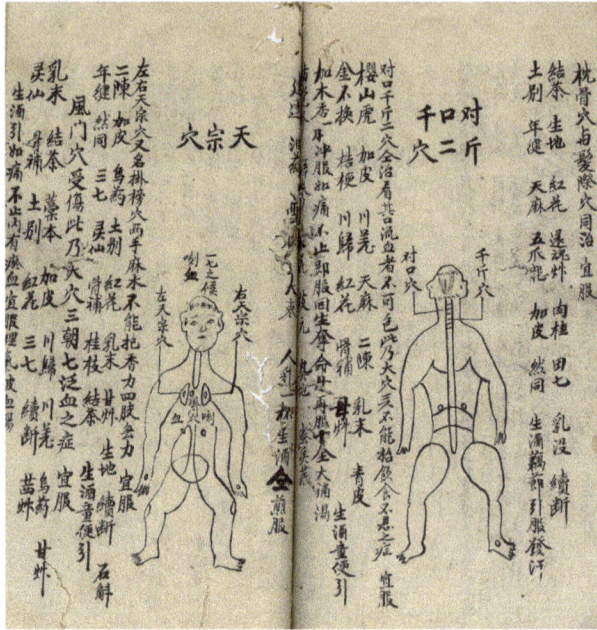

SURVEY OF CONTENTS: This volume appears to include two different texts, although from the wording of the preface the book's two parts should be two *juan* of one single text. The preface dated 1890 states: 吾友邵子勤俊，業究軒岐，術精盧扁，斷筋折骨，運藥即痊，石毒金瘡，傅膏輒癒。既得異人傳授，遂與良相同功。由是苦心考究，蒼（薈）萃羣方，輯成□卷。......展而讀之，見其論症製方，皆切切多有深意。且繪圖以分部位，使後學一見瞭然。......光緒十六年庚寅仲夏通家弟南海羅汝霖敬書.

The preface is followed by a table of contents. The first two paragraphs are Cha zheng guan mai can yi yong yao lun 察症觀脈參宜用藥論, "On examing the signs of disease and inspecting the vessels to use medication in an appropriate manner", and Die da sun shang yong yao lun 跌打損傷用藥論, "On the use of medication for injuries resulting from falls and blows". The following is a listing of 94 pharmaceutical recipes, different from the table of contents which lists 109 entries. The bibliography *Zhong guo zhong yi gu ji zong mu* 中國中醫古籍總目 has no records of a book written by Shao Qinjun 邵勤俊 on traumatology. The present text focusses on pharmaceutical treatments of ruptured sinews and bone fractures. It includes numerous illustrations of the human body with the names and locations of "holes", 穴 *xue*, and an explanation, not seen in any other text, of the significance of injury caused by blows against these locations.

This section is followed by a second with its own table of contents, including the following paragraphs:

認真辨傷法 看症定生死法 準定擒拿定生死總論 八死症要訣 分傷輕重讚 定穴道受傷生死時刻讚 擒拿運手（通關）妙訣 擒（拿）走手推法(論) 周 身穴道尺寸論 擒拿開竅妙訣 側面點穴重傷名 七十（二）式擒拿妙訣總章 初動搞（擒）總決 二用總手訣 三擒後（移）定生死訣 擒分陰陽雙單訣 擒 拿定度秘訣 擒拿秘訣總手論 凡人周身六道尺寸訣 擒拿用藥論 回生奪命丹 真人活命飲 平胃開中散 理氣破血散 活命和中散 擒拿救命死回生訣 均氣 散 七仙丹 接骨定痛麻藥丹 接骨還原丹 接骨還服藥方 金槍還原丹 鐵扇散 開手發蒙秘訣 擒拿用藥論 十不治症.

However, the actual contents following the table of contents do not entirely agree with the list given above. Preceding the first paragraph on 認真辨傷法, additional paragraphs include the following: 各穴受傷用藥論、鳥槍沙子入 肉方、箭鏃鉛子入肉方、銃子入肉方、自刎急救方、打出眼睛、接骨神方 東平展子明傳.

Following the final paragraph "Ten incurable illness conditions", Shi bu zhi zheng 十不治症, listed in the table of contents, an additional paragraph concluding the main text is: "Illustrated patterns for a treatment with pharmaceutical drugs of all [needle insertion] holes where injury was inflicted", Ge xue shou shang yong yao tu shi 各穴受傷用藥圖式. The locations where harm is received illustrated and discussed here are the following: 太陽、迎香、天 庭耳寸穴、血倉咽喉穴、玉堂缺盆穴、心窩左右乳下穴、中腕穴、期門 穴、氣海膀胱穴、髮際穴、對口千斤二穴、天宗穴、肺腧心腧穴、命門腎 俞穴、膀胱尾底穴、掛膀委陽穴、開空穴、太陽穴、飛燕入洞、右飛燕入 洞、脾骨穴、掛膀穴、鳳尾穴、印堂穴、鼻樑穴、咽喉正穴、牙腮牙骨、 命空穴、肚角穴、童子骨、對口穴、背漏穴、胃脘、心窩穴、中管穴、肚 臍穴、膀胱穴、胃脘穴、左邊氣門大穴、左邊氣血乳下二指、淨瓶穴、鳳 翅盆穴、左右將臺穴、腰骨腰眼穴、尾底穴、下竅封門穴、膝蓋穴、寸關 尺穴、背脊穴、腳背穴、雙鳳朝陽穴、仙人套印、麒麟環跳二穴. Each of these illustrations is followed by advice on suitable pharmaceutical therapy, often interspersed with exorcistic approaches, such as oral and written spells. They are not listed in the table of contents, and were possibly inserted by a later copyist of the text.

Although the contents of this volume are very rich, it is unclear to which tradition it may belong. It requires further research.

\*\*\*

| TITLE: | *Shang han she jian* 傷寒舌鑒, Harm caused by cold as re-flected by the tongue |
| --- | --- |
| ID: | 8846 |
| CONTENTS: | Tongue diagnosis |
| APPEARANCE: | Ancient manuscript. Edges minimally damaged. Paper quality quite old. Cover prepared from waste paper with notes on pharmaceutical recipes. Inscription: Shang han ke 傷寒科. Main text carefully copied. Excellent calligraphy. |
| BINDING: | Thread |
| MEASURE: | 19.8 x. 11.3 |
| TITLE PAGE: | No. |
| NO. OF PAGES: | 70 |
| L.P. /CH.L: | 9 x 8 |
| LAYOUT: | Each page with four horizontal lines separating three sections with data below a broad empty upper margin and a |

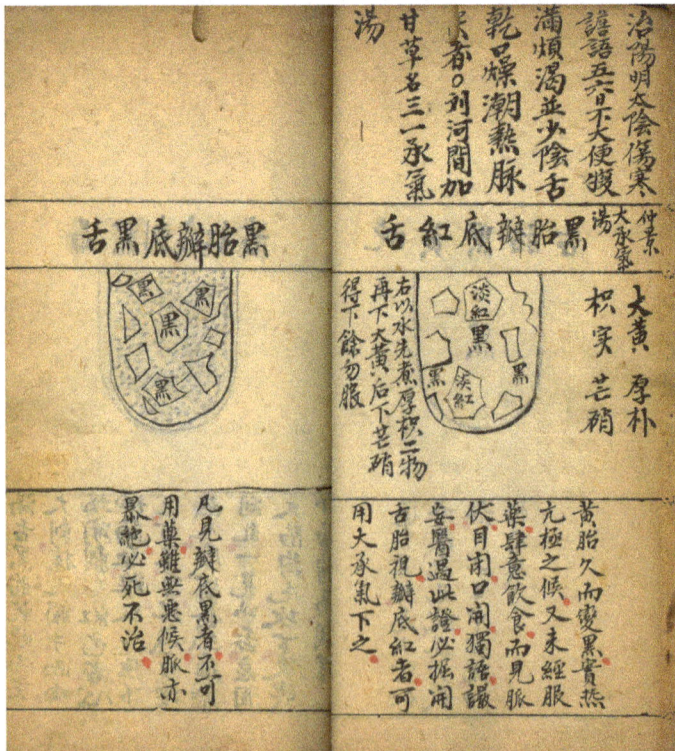

narrow empty lower section. The uppermost data section provides a designation of a specific appearance of the tongue. The section below provides a b/w drawing of the tongue in question. The lowermost data section provides an explanatory comment.

AUTHOR AND YEAR OF TEXT:

Qing. Zhang Deng 張登, 1668

YEAR OF COPY: No Qing dynasty taboos observed. Republican era.

SURVEY OF CONTENTS: This volume is on tongue diagnosis. It is a selective copy of the Qing era author Zhang Deng's *Shang han she jian* 傷寒舌鑒 with a discussion of the significance of 120 different tongue appearances. A first section 白胎舌總論 is missing in the present copy; also, at its end the final page showing and discussing a "curled and shortened tongue in pregnant women harmed by cold", 孕婦傷寒卷短舌, is missing. The illustrations of the tongues and the text written below them are quite accurate. This is a good handwritten copy of the *Shang han she jian* 傷寒舌鑒.

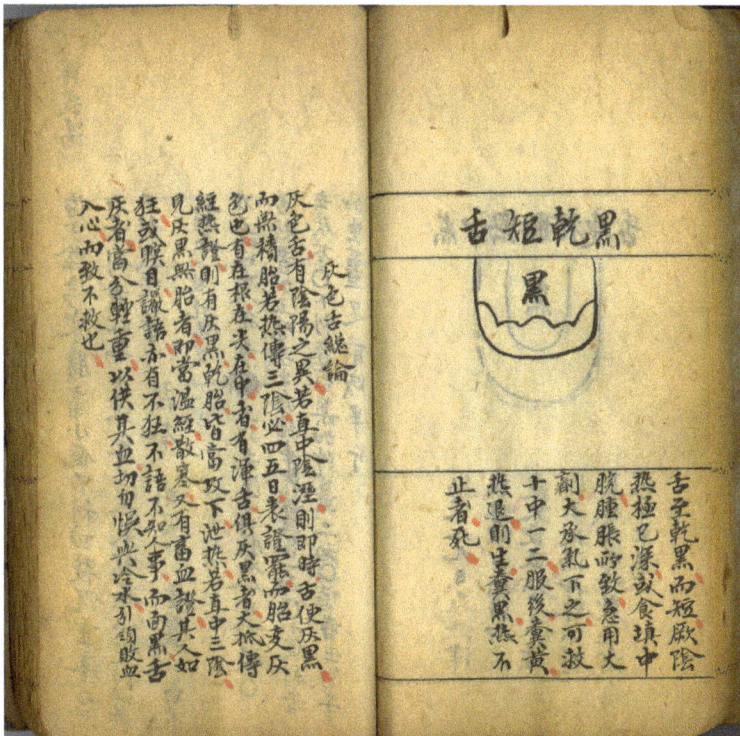

*** 

TITLE:            *Xiao'er tui na fang mai huo ying mi zhi quan shu* 小兒推拿
                  方脈活嬰秘旨全書, Book on secret instructions to keep
                  infants alive by means of pediatric push-and-pull massage
                  recipes.

ID:               8847

CONTENTS:         Pediatrics

APPEARANCE:       Ancient manuscript. Original front cover missing. Blank
                  page added as cover by later person, with repeated inscrip-
                  tion 推拿全書. Handwriting rather deficient.

BINDING:          Thread

MEASURE:          18.2 x 12.7

TITLE PAGE:       No

NO. OF PAGES:     75

L.P. /CH.L:       11 x approx. 19

LAYOUT:           Paper with vertical red lines. Writing does not follow the
                  given columns. 11 x approx. 19. The writing diverges from

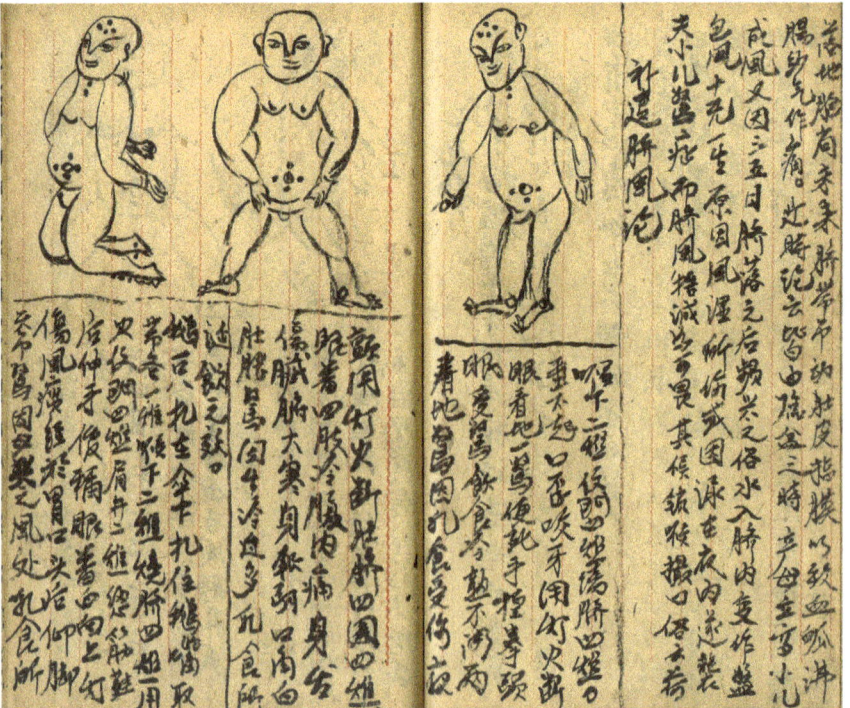

traditional handwriting. It begins on the left and continues in vertical columns to the right. When closed, the edge with the binding points to the left.

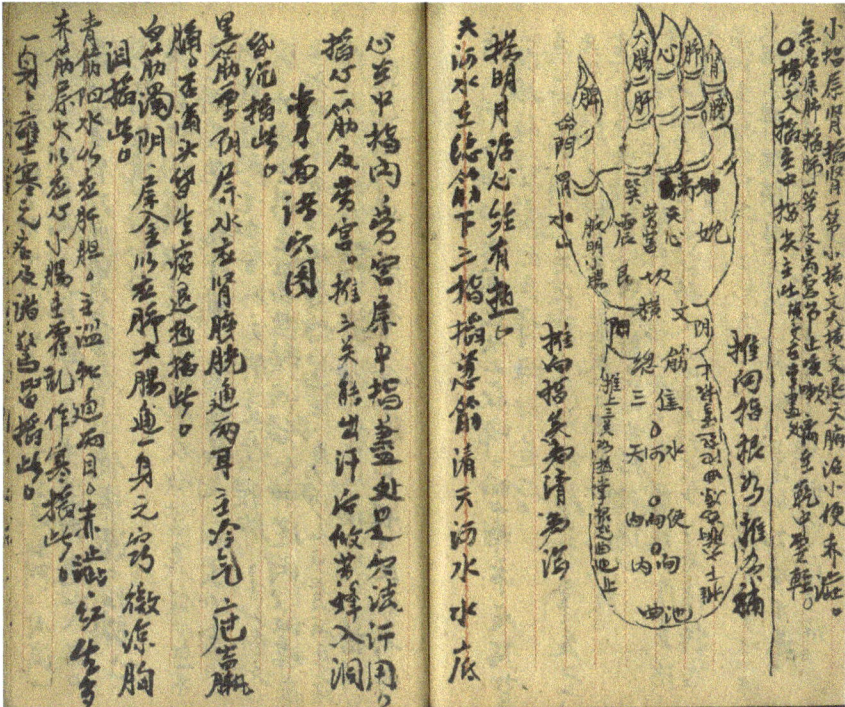

AUTHOR AND YEAR OF TEXT:

Ming, Gong Tingxian 龚廷贤; amended by Yao Guozhen 姚国桢.

YEAR OF COPY:    Recent copy. Around 1950

SURVEY OF CONTENTS: The main text begins on the first page with the title of the original text: *Xin ke xiao'er tui na fang mai huo ying mi zhi quan shu* 新刻小兒推拿方脈活嬰秘旨全書, with additional information on the author: 金溪龙（龔）云林, Gong Yunlin from Jinxi, the Imperial Physician Yao Guozhen 姚国桢who amended and edited the text, as well as on a further person who had the book printed. The text includes many abbreviated characters, further indicating that it was copied in more recent times.

***

| | |
|---|---|
| TITLE: | *Jiu ji liang fang* 救急良方, Good recipes for help in urgent cases |
| ID: | 8848 |
| CONTENTS: | Pharmaceutical recipes |
| APPEARANCE: | Ancient manuscript. Coarse paper quality. Handwriting quite fine. Blue cover made from bast fibre of the paper mulberry paper, with a red label providing the inscription: 民國拾陸年新春立草料飯賬綹. Hence this is not the original cover of this book; it was used for another manuscript before. The back of the front page is inscribed with a pharmaceutical recipe. |
| BINDING: | Paper spills |
| MEASURE: | 14.8 x 28.0 |
| TITLE PAGE: | The 2nd page is the original title page. It has a red inscription: "Good recipes for help in urgent cases", *Jiu ji liang fang* 救急良方, and a further inscription with black ink: 民國弎 |

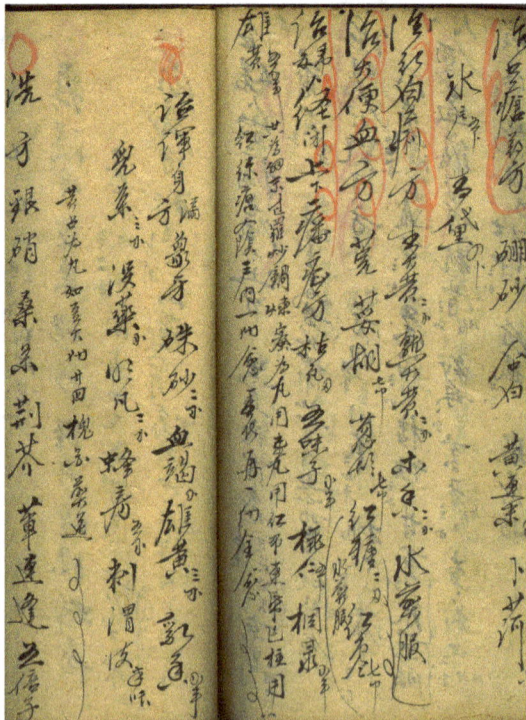

拾弍年龍月立醫按以共肆拾叁賬, "Republic, 33rd year, *long* ("dragon") month, [I have] written down these medical notes, all together 43 paragraphs".

NO. OF PAGES:          48

L.P. /CH.L:            6-7 x approx. 18

LAYOUT:                No lines, no frames

AUTHOR AND YEAR OF TEXT:

                      Unknown

YEAR OF COPY:          As noted on the title page, the volume was written in 1944.

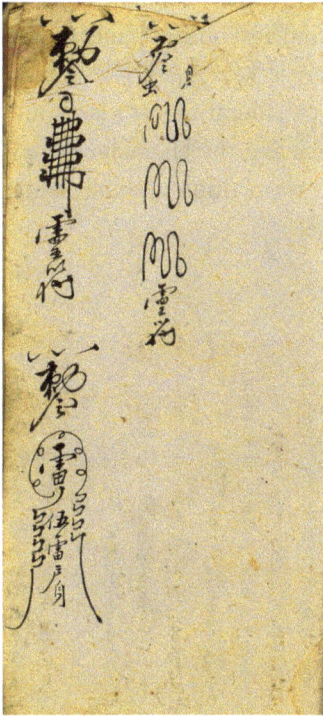

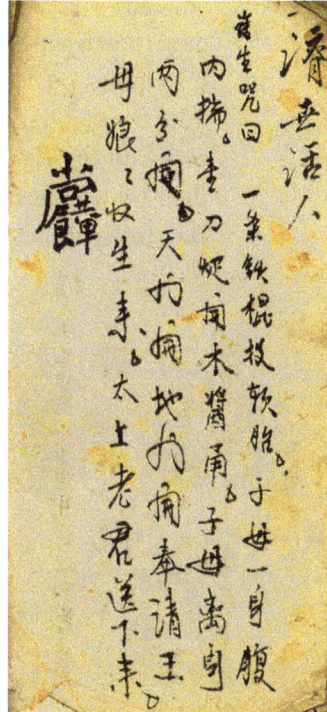

SURVEY OF CONTENTS: This is a record of 261 pharmaceutical recipes in a rather hasty writing. Two additional pages of smaller size have been inserted and bound with the main text of the volume. The recipes are for all types of therapeutic indications; their listing follows no apparent order. Presumably, they were recorded over time as the copyist came to know of them. They are mostly well known recipes from printed books, including patent prescriptions. Only a few are single substance recipes as used by the common people. Towards the end of the volume the copyist listed a few exorcistic therapies.

\*\*\*

| | |
|---|---|
| TITLE: | (*Wai ke shi san fang* 外科十三方, Thirteen recipes from external medicine) |
| ID: | 8849 |
| CONTENTS: | External medicine |
| APPEARANCE: | Simple, crude ancient manuscript. Brittle paper turned brown. |
| BINDING: | Original paper spills still in place. Later new thread binding added with new front cover (white cotton paper) and title page (tough paper made from bast fibre of paper mulberry). Inscription on front cover: 活人妙方/于溥澤. Interior of front cover and title page with four prints of a large, circular seal with the eight trigrams and the character *hong* 鴻 in their center. The main text was written in small characters. Handwriting above average. |
| MEASURE: | 18.3 x 13.1 |

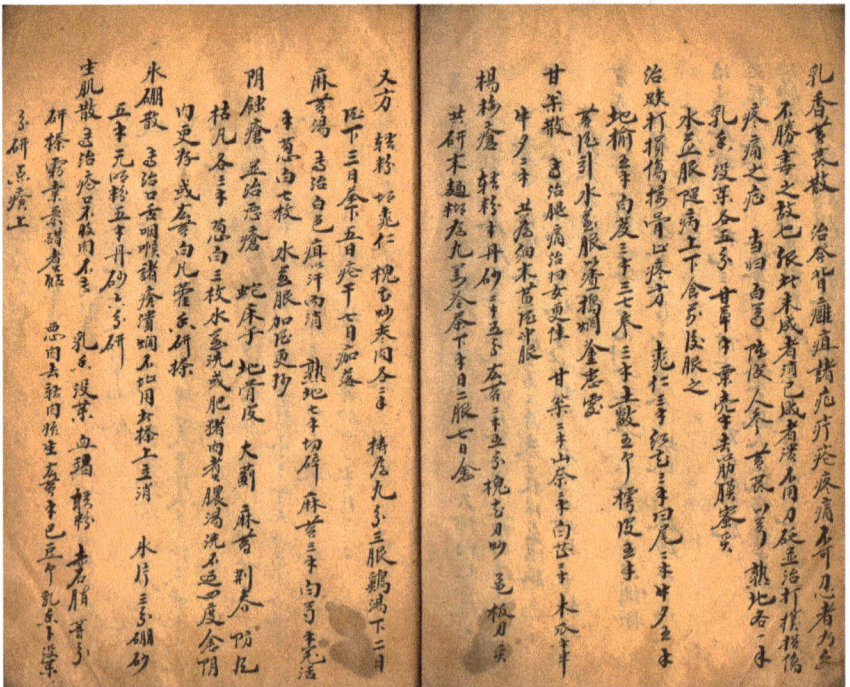

TITLE PAGE:      Later added. Inscription: 救世仙方/葉天氏云/救人一命鴻福齊天

NO. OF PAGES:    22

L.P. /CH.L:    12 x approx. 24

LAYOUT:    No lines, no frames

AUTHOR AND YEAR OF TEXT:

    Possibly Qing, Guan Xiandeng 管先登.

YEAR OF COPY:    No Qing dynasty taboos observed. Republican era.

SURVEY OF CONTENTS: The beginning of the original volume is missing. The remaining text shows a characteristic structure. It employs a question and answer dialogue to explain pathological conditions encountered in external medicine. For example: 何為痰核、瘰癧？答曰：大為痰核，小為瘰癧, "what are phlegm seeds, and scrofula? Answer: large ones are phlegm seeds; small ones are scrofula", etc. A comparison of this text section with Chinese medicine texts accessible through electronic means shows that it is similar to the contents of a section Shi ba wen da 十八問答, "18 Questions and Answers", in the final chapter of the *Wai ke shi san fang kao* 外科十三方考, "An examination of 13 recipes from External Medicine", of 1947 compiled by a more recent author Zhang Jueren 張覺人. Still the present text appears to have omitted some passages and added others. The recipes *ma liang gao* 麻凉膏 and *xun xi tang* 熏洗湯 copied here can also be found in the *Wai ke shi san fang kao* 外科十三方考. That is, there must have been some link between the present volume and the *Wai ke shi san fang kao* 外科十三方考. A book with similar title is a work compiled by the Qing author Guan Xiandeng 管先登, with the title 管氏外科十三方, *Guan shi wai ke shi san fang* of 1855. However, this book is quite difficult to access today, so we had no opportunity of inspecting its contents. Hence we can only hypothesize whether the present manuscript volume is related to this book.

In its final section, this volume records several tens of pharmaceutical recipes, all of them regularly used in external medicine. However, their origin is unclear. There are no recipes transmitted among the common people.

***

TITLE:                 *Si bai wei* 肆百味, Four hundred substances
ID:                    8850
CONTENTS:              Materia medica
APPEARANCE:            Account-book size ancient manuscript. Margins and edges
                       slightly damaged. Fine handwriting. Cover: thin writing pa-
                       per made from bamboo, with inscription: 肆百味/張近義/
                       丁亥年拾月廿三立
BINDING:               Thread
MEASURE:               14.0 x 23.4
TITLE PAGE:            No
NO. OF PAGES:          28
L.P. /CH.L:            13 x approx. 7
LAYOUT:                No lines, no frames
AUTHOR AND YEAR OF TEXT:
                       Zhang Jinyi 張近義, 1947
YEAR OF COPY:          1947

SURVEY OF CONTENTS: This is a list of approximately 700 pharmaceutical drugs with their major therapeutic effects. This listing is special in that the names of the drugs are not those given in pharmaceutical literature. Rather they are written here with their specifications (such as "best quality", or "harvested in XYZ") as they are prescribed by physicians. Also, their sequence does not follow the first characters of each drug name, but the final character. This way all drug names ending with the character *hua* 花, "flower", are listed together, as are those ending with the character *cao* 草, "herb". This type of ordering the names of substances is frequently found in the pharmaceutical business. It helps to bring together substances of the same type. However, such a system is not entirely coherent. For example, the final character *zi* 子 in the name *nü zhen zi* 女貞子 refers to a fruit. In the name *mu bie zi* 木鱉子 it refers to seeds. In *wu pei zi* 五倍子 it refers to botanical galls. In *jing tu zi* 淨土子 it refers to the brown iron ore kernels found in it. In *lu bian zi* 鹿鞭子 it refers to a deer's penis. In *tian kui zi* 天葵子 it refers to the root of the plant, and in *yan fu zi* 鹽附子 it refers to the root of a plant immersed in brine.

The present manuscript is evidence of the classification of and effects assigned to pharmaceutical substances as was common until the Republican era.

***

| | |
|---|---|
| TITLE: | *Chong jiao tang tou ge jue* 重校湯頭歌訣, Newly edited *Tang tou ge jue*. |
| ID: | 8851 |
| CONTENTS: | Pharmaceutical recipes |
| APPEARANCE: | Simple ancient manuscript volume. Careful handwriting. Average calligraphy. |
| BINDING: | Paper spills |
| MEASURE: | 21.0 x 10.8 |
| TITLE PAGE: | Inscription from left to right: 重校湯頭歌訣/民國叁年/王五則誦 |
| NO. OF PAGES: | 22 |
| L.P. /CH.L: | 6 x 19 |
| LAYOUT: | No lines, no frames |
| AUTHOR AND YEAR OF TEXT: | |
| | Qing. Wang Ang 汪昂. |
| YEAR OF COPY: | 1914 |

SURVEY OF CONTENTS: This is an excerpt copy from the Qing author Wang Ang's 汪昂 work *Tang tou ge jue* 湯頭歌訣. The text is not divided; it lists 58 recipes beginning with recipes assumed "to supplement", *bu yi* 補益, and ending

with recipes assumed "to order qi", *li qi* 理氣. At the conclusion of the volume
the author added two notes. The first was a warning concerning ancient dosage amounts given with the recipes: "The dosage amounts requested in these
recipes are uneven. Some make use of 3 *qian* 錢or 5 *qian*, others make use of
four or five *liang* 兩, or six to seven *liang*. For example, *da cheng qi tang* 大承
氣湯, "major decoction to uphold the qi". The one ingredient *da huang* 大黃 is
used with up to four *liang*. Nowadays, certainly no one would dare to use four
*liang*. Only four to five *qian* may be used. Or another example: of *ban xia* 半夏
the dosis each time is half a *sheng* 半升. This too is not to be relied upon. ... As
for the dosages of pharmaceutical substances recommended in this *Tang tou
ge jue*, at the time of their usage a dosage recommended in terms of *liang* may
be employed today as *qian*. It is absolutely impossible to use several *liang* of
one single substance. The dosages must be deliberated at the very moment [of
therapy]. Watch this! Watch this!" The final note identified the copyist of the
present volume: "This volume was prepared by Comrade Wang Quanwu 王全

五, at the time of his affiliation with the Association for the Protection of the People." The handwriting of this note is inferior and unlike that of the main text.

*** 

| | |
|---|---|
| TITLE: | (*Tie da shang xue jiu zhi fa* 跌打傷穴救治法. Patterns for the rescue and therapy [of patients] harmed at [needle insertion] holes by falls and blows.) |
| ID: | 8852 |
| CONTENTS: | Bonesetting, traumatology |
| APPEARANCE: | Ancient manuscript with a red-brown cover of tough paper made from the bast fiber of paper mulberry. Faint inscription: 寶信本全傳/羅有絲. Inside of back cover with inscription: 羅有絲. The paper is rather crude. It looks as if an account book had been given a new binding. Average calligraphy. |
| BINDING: | Thread |

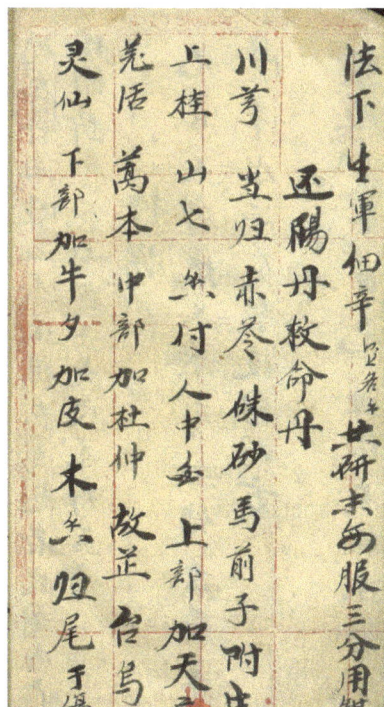

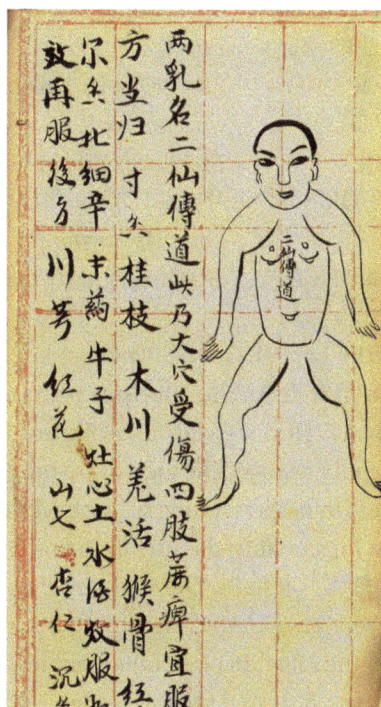

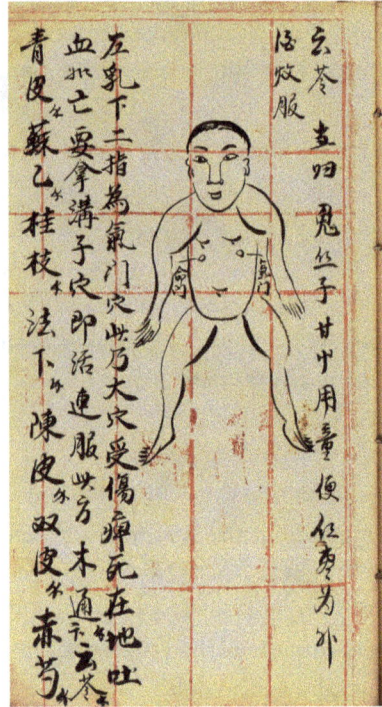

MEASURE:　　　　　26.5 x 15.5
TITLE PAGE:　　　　Blank
NO. OF PAGES:　　　32 plus 2 pp blank
L.P. /CH.L:　　　　>8 x approx. 20
LAYOUT:　　　　　Red lines and margins.
AUTHOR AND YEAR OF TEXT:
　　　　　　　　　Qing. Anonymous
YEAR OF COPY:　　No Qing dynasty taboos observed. Republican era.

SURVEY OF CONTENTS: The first line of this volume states Quan shen tui na jue fa 全身推拿訣法, "Decisive patterns of push-and-pull massage for the entire body." However, the following text is only marginally related to *tuina* push-and-pull massage. The focus is on traumatology and pharmaceutical therapies to treat injuries resulting from blows directed at specific "holes", *xue* 穴, on the body. Presumably, the title of the original writing was *Tie da shang xue jiu zhi fa* 跌打傷穴救治法. The contents are as follows:

A section with the title Quan shen tui na jue fa 全身推拿訣法 relates how to judge the location of an injury on the basis of the pathological signs following an injury. A second section Yao fang 藥方 lists 6 pharmaceutical recipes. This is followed by three drawings of the human body. The first two show a complete human body indicating its sections. The third is devoted to injuries received at the Yellow Bees hole, *huang feng xue* 黃蜂穴, with the subsequent text detailing the pathological signs resulting from an injury there. The text advises to first manipulate the so called ditch hole, *gou zi* 溝子穴, and then to ingest liquid medication and apply *tui na*-massage. This is followed by illustrated text on the consequences of harm received at the location of further "holes", i.e., *gua pang xue* 掛膀穴, *feng wei* 鳳尾, *ren zhong xue* 人中穴, *yan kong xue* 咽空穴, *ya bei ya sai* 牙背牙腮, *yan hou* 咽喉, *ding quan feng bo* 頂圈·鳳膊, *jiang tai xue* 將台穴, *ren kong xue* 人空穴, *tian ping zhen* 天平針, *xin xia zhong wan* 心下中脘, *du ji da ke xue* 肚臍大客穴, *pang guang* 膀胱, *liang ru* 兩乳 (*er xian chuan dao* 二仙傳道), *qi men xue* 氣門穴, *er ru xia zhi* 二乳下指 (*xue qi* 血氣, *xue tan* 血痰), *xue wan jing ping* 血脘淨瓶 (below the soft ribs on the left side), *du jiao* 肚角, *ming gong xue* 命宮穴 (below the ribs on the right side), *pen xuan* 盆弦 (abdominal egde on the right) *feng bo gu tong zi gu* 鳳膊骨·童子骨, *xi gai xi gen* 膝蓋·膝眼, *jiao bei* 腳背, *dui kou xue* 對口穴, *bei gou ren kong xue* 背漏人空穴, *yao yan* 腰眼. This is followed by advice on further such pharmaceutical treatment, but without illustrations: *tong hu di lou ji wei jie gu shou shang fang* 銅壺滴漏及尾結骨受傷方, "recipe for harm received at the 'dripping clepsydra' and tailbone", *feng men xue feng yin xue shou shang fang* 鳳門穴鳳陰穴受傷方, "recipe for harm received at the *feng men* and *feng yin* holes", *bu jin shou shang fang* 布筋受傷方, "recipe for harm received by the sinews", *feng dao jin yao fang* 逢刀斧藥方, "pharmaceutical recipe for [injuries] inflicted by knife or hatchet". Many of the "holes" listed, and the suggested therapy patterns, are not found in printed books.

*** 

| | |
|---|---|
| TITLE: | *Hou ke zhi zhang* 喉科指掌, A guide through laryngology. |
| ID: | 8853 |
| CONTENTS: | Laryngology |
| APPEARANCE: | Beautiful ancient manuscript volume. Green fabric pasted on a paper cover. No damage whatsoever. Remnants of a red title paper label, with only one readable character left: 不. Back cover with 4-characters seal: 謙益公製 |
| BINDING: | Special type of thread-binding. Edges with a caps lock. |
| MEASURE: | 23.8 x 16.6 |

TITLE PAGE:         No
NO. OF PAGES:       35
L.P. /CH.L:         10 x approx. 17
LAYOUT:             Red lines and frames, as in account books.
AUTHOR AND YEAR OF TEXT:
                    Qing. Zhang Zongliang 張宗良, 1757. Copyist: Qian Yigong
                    謙益公
YEAR OF COPY:       Paper quality, nature of ink, and failure to observe Qing dy-
                    nasty taboos suggest that this volume was written during
                    the Republican period.

SURVEY OF CONTENTS: This manuscript is on laryngology. The first line of the
text states: 七十二症主治： 六味湯. This is followed by a list of throat ailments
beginning with 咽喉門一·簾珠喉 and concluding with 左陰瘡七、右陰瘡八.
Each throat ailment is given a separate paragraph, with an illustration above
and an explanatory text plus pharmaceutical recipe(s) below. This is a selective
copy of four *juan* of the Qing author Zhang Zongliang's 張宗良 work *Hou ke
zhi zhang* 喉科指掌, including the sections beginning with Yan hou men 咽喉
門 of *juan* 3 and concluding with the section Za hou men 雜喉門 of *juan* 6. To
this was added a copy of several pharmaceutical recipes from the *Hou ke zhi
zhang*'s 喉科指掌 section Jing xuan yingyong zhu fang 精選應用諸方, "Care-

fully chosen recipes for appropriate application" in its 2nd *juan*. This includes a Shi ba wei shen yao 十八味神藥, "Divine medication of 18 substances", as well as several pharmaceutical recipes for diverse therapeutic indications that were not listed in the *Hou ke zhi zhang* 喉科指掌.

***

| | |
|---|---|
| TITLE: | (*Dou tai shi chuang yang jing yan quan shu* 竇太師瘡瘍經驗全書, Complete writings by Grand Teacher Dou on his experience with lesions and ulcers) |
| ID: | 8854 |
| CONTENTS: | External medicine |
| APPEARANCE: | 4 ancient manuscript volumes with margins slightly damaged, and covers missing. Average handwriting. Title page is cover now. |
| BINDING: | Thread |
| MEASURE: | 22.5 x 13.0 |
| TITLE PAGE: | First vol. title page with red inscription from left to right: 手腕發背疔毒圖說症方計柒拾條/嘉慶拾柒年十二月十三日立. The first line from the left手腕發背疔毒圖說症方計柒拾條 repeated by later hand with fountain pen in blue. Second vol.: cover missing. Inscription on title page: 腿膝足倍及諸瘤圖方計捌拾條/嘉慶拾柒年拾弎月十三日立. Also, black inscription: 痔漏藥/天慶公記. Third vol. with red inscription on title page: 痘瘡形症圖說湯論治法/嘉慶拾柒年拾弎月十三日立. Fourth vol. with red inscription on title page: 用藥脈訣五臟□□□決生死治法/嘉慶拾柒年拾弎月十三日/瓚卿. |
| NO. OF PAGES: | Vol. 1: 52. Vol. 2: 38. Vol. 3: 38. Vol. 4: 65 |
| L.P. /CH.L: | 7 x approx. 32 |
| LAYOUT: | No lines, no frames |
| AUTHOR AND YEAR OF TEXT: | |
| | Ming. Dou Menglin 竇夢麟 with later addenda. |
| YEAR OF COPY: | Characters 玄 and 淡 written without observing Qing dynasty taboos. The date given on the cover, *jiaqing* 17th year, is 1812. Nevertheless, these volumes may have been written as late as in the Republican era. |

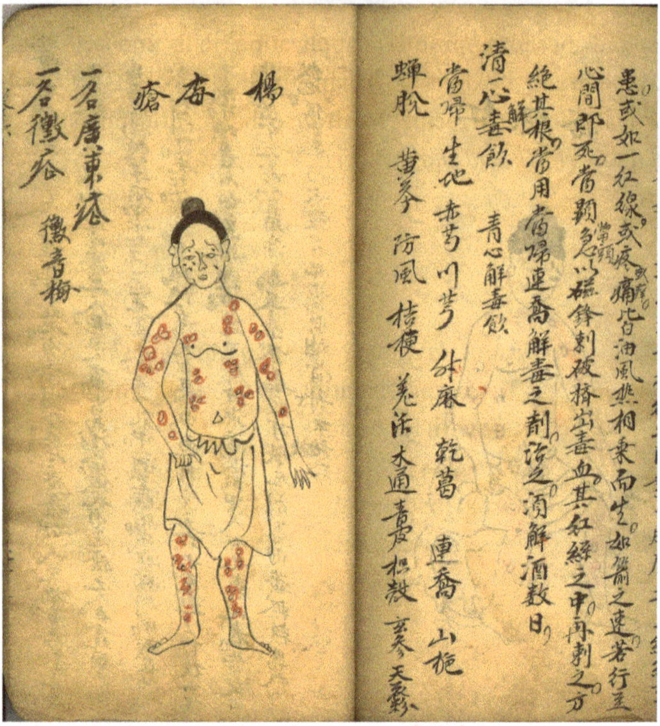
楊梅瘡
一名廣東瘡
一名徽瘡
清心解毒飲

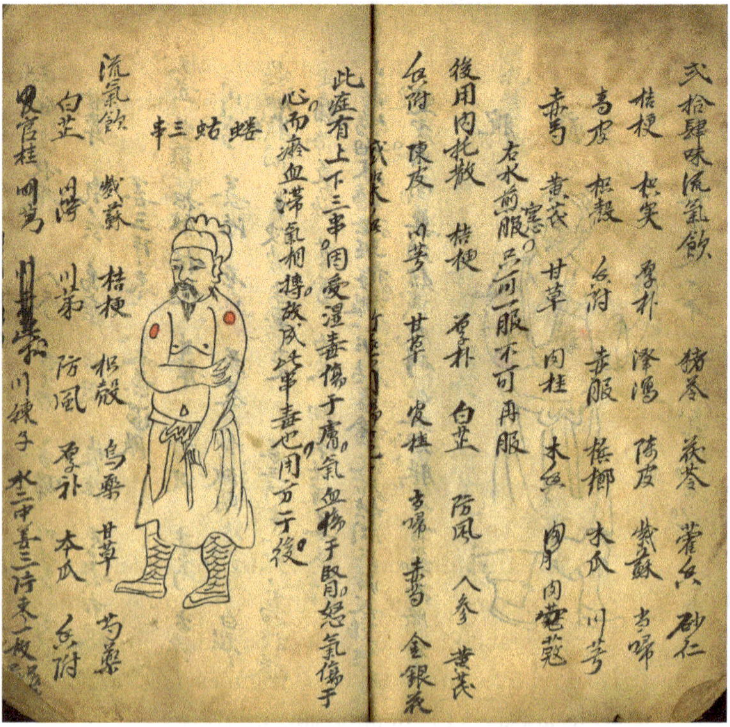
貳拾肆味流氣飲
蝲蛄三串
流氣飲

SURVEY OF CONTENTS: Two volumes are copies of the Ming author Dou Men-glin's 竇夢麟 *Chong ke Dou tai shi chuang yang jing yan quan shu* 重刻竇太師瘡瘍經驗全書. The first volume begins with a Juan zhi si mu lu 卷之肆目錄, "Table of contents of *juan* 4", with all sections listed from "Poison [erupting] in the palm of the hand", Shou xin du 手心毒, to "Fish belly-type pin-illness", Yu qi ding 魚臍疗. The second volume begins with the section He xi feng 鶴膝風,, "Crane knee wind", and ends with Zhu liu 諸瘤, "Various tumors". This is the sixth *juan* of the *Chong ke Dou tai shi chuang yang jing yan quan shu* 重刻竇太师疮疡经验全书. Hence these are only two of the 13 *juan* of the original text. The third vol. has 宋竇太師瘡瘍經驗全書□□小兒痘瘡/圖論方. This is the eighth *juan* of the original book. The fourth volume has 宋竇太師瘡瘍經驗全書/炮製法、用附子說......"。This is the tenth *juan* of the original text. Following the table of contents the entire text of Shi chuan mi fang pao zhi fa 世傳秘方炮製法 is added.

The *Dou tai shi chuang yang jing yan quan shu* 竇太師瘡瘍經驗全書 was compiled by the Song author Dou Jie 竇傑 (Zisheng 子聲; Hanqing 漢卿). It was further enlarged by Dou Menglin 竇夢麟, and published in the 3rd year of the Ming dynasty reign period *longqing* 隆慶, i.e., 1569. *Juan* 1 through 4 have illustrations showing pathological conditions of the throat, teeth, and tongue;

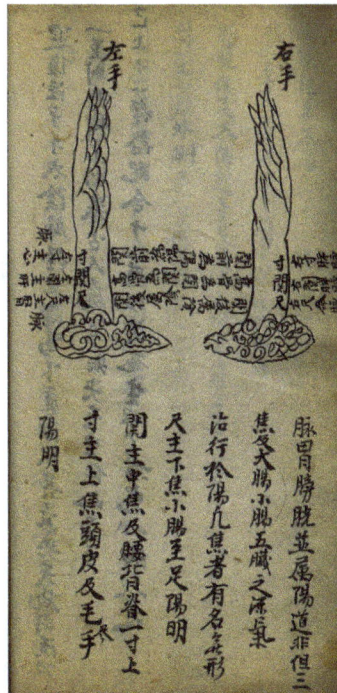

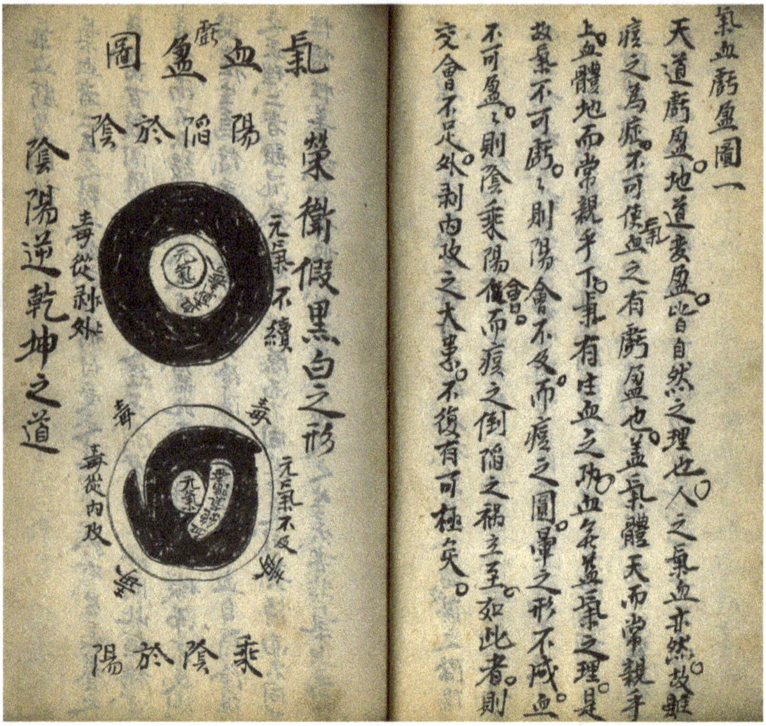
氣血虧盈圖一
天道虧盈。地道變盈。皆自然之理也。人之氣血亦然。故雖
痘之爲症。不可使氣血之有虧盈也。蓋氣體天而常親乎
上。血體地而常親乎下。氣有生血之功。血無益氣之理。是
故氣不可虧。虧則陽會不及。而痘之圓暈之形不成。血
不可盈。盈則陰乘陽位。而痘之倒陷之禍立至。如此者。則
交會不足。外剝內攻之大患。不復有可救矣。
氣血虧盈圖
榮衛假黑白之形
陽陷於陰
元氣不續
毒從剝外
元氣不及
毒從內攻
陰乘於陽
陰陽逆乾坤之道

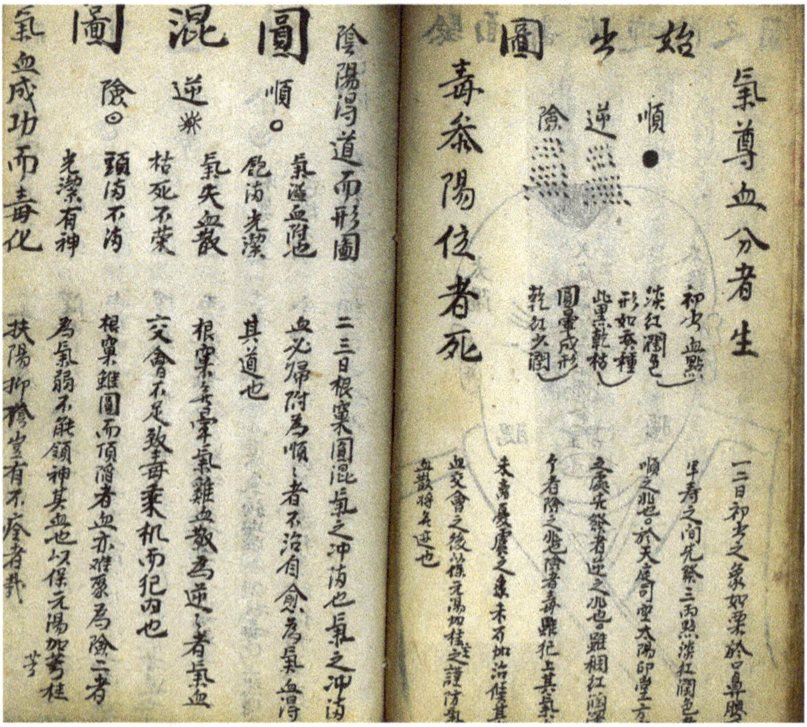
氣尊血分者生
始出圖
毒參陽位者死
順
逆
險
陰陽得道而形圓
圓混圖
順。
逆
險
氣血成功而毒化

impediment illness (*ju* 疽) affecting chest and face; obstruction illness with poison (*yong du* 癰毒) affecting chest, flanks, lower back, and abdomen; pin-illness (*ding* 疔) affecting the wrists and effusing on the back. *Juan* 5 through 9 offer illustrations on pathological conditions of "poison in the region of relief" (*bian du* 便毒), and "bone impediment-illness" (*gu ju* 骨疽), all types of tumors affecting the legs, knees, and feet; *da ma feng* 大麻風, leprosy; *gan du* 疳毒, *gan*-illness poison; and *dou chuang* 痘瘡, pox sores, as well as advice on moxa cauterization, petty surgery, and on medication to dissolve poison. *Juan* 10 through 13 include sections such as Yong yao mai jue wu zang tu 用藥脈訣五臟圖, Shen zhi za bing qi fang 神治雜病奇方, Guai zheng ji xiao er za zheng fang 怪症及小兒雜症方, Zheng chuang zong shuo huo jian zhi yan fang 癥瘡總說或間治驗方法, and Yi ji 宜忌. The present manuscript volumes offer only a selection of the treatises found in the original text.

***

| | |
|---|---|
| TITLE: | (*Yao fang za chao* 藥方雜抄, A copy of miscellaneous pharmaceutical recipes) |
| ID: | 8855 |
| CONTENTS: | Pharmaceutical recipes |
| APPEARANCE: | Simple ancient manuscript volume. Average handwriting. Cover made of paper mulberry paper; no title. Inscription: 雪山會奚六千六百八十五人, unrelated to the contents of the manuscript. |
| BINDING: | Paper spills |
| MEASURE: | 27.5 x 14.9 |
| TITLE PAGE: | No |
| NO. OF PAGES: | 11 |
| L.P. /CH.L: | 6 x >34 |
| LAYOUT: | No lines, no frames |
| AUTHOR AND YEAR OF TEXT: | Unknown |
| YEAR OF COPY: | Recent paper quality. Fresh ink color. Republican period or later. |

SURVEY OF CONTENTS: This is a listing of 53 pharmaceutical recipes mostly from the realms of gynecology and external medicine. Among the gynecological recipes are those "to open the bones in the case of difficult birth", *nan chan kai gu* 難產開骨, "to keep the fetus", *cun tai* 存胎, "a method to end fertility", *duan zi fa* 斷子法, "recipe for medication to be ingested for stimulating delivery", *xia chan chi yao fang* 下產吃藥方, "recipe specifically designed for abortion", *zhuan zhi da tai fang* 專治打胎方 (with *cai zi gan* 菜籽杆, "rapeseed stems", *ji ji zi* 極極籽, "field thistle seeds", 雀臥蛋, "trailing spurge", *ban mao* 斑毛, "mylabris beetle"). The dosage quantities are specified with the *hua ma* 花碼 counting system. Also, there is yet another extremely rarely seen counting system whereby to a character *shi* 十 ("ten") dots are added to the upper left edge. The details of this system are unknown to us. The recipes include one "recipe for children's and women's brickbed-wetting", *er nü niao kan fang* 兒女尿炕方, with an extremely rare therapeutic approach: "*Xiong huang* 雄黃, 3 *qian,* and two knots of aged onions 老蔥乙結 are to be ground to pulp. The pulp is placed on the navel of the abdomen and covered with cotton. This is then tied to the lower back with a piece of cloth to be left for one night. One hundred applications will result in one hundred successes."

*** 

| | |
|---|---|
| TITLE: | *Bai li yao fang* 百例藥方, One hundred selected pharmaceutical recipes. |
| ID: | 8856 |
| CONTENTS: | Pharmaceutical recipes |
| APPEARANCE: | Thin, simple manuscript volume. Inscription on cover with fountain pen in abbreviated characters: 百例药方. Average calligraphy; irregular writing. |
| BINDING: | Paper spills |
| MEASURE: | 22.0 x 14.0 |
| TITLE PAGE: | No |
| NO. OF PAGES: | 12 |
| L.P. /CH.L: | 7 x. approx. 29 |
| LAYOUT: | No lines, no frames |
| AUTHOR AND YEAR OF TEXT: | Unknown |
| YEAR OF COPY: | Recent paper quality. Fresh ink color. Republican period or later. |

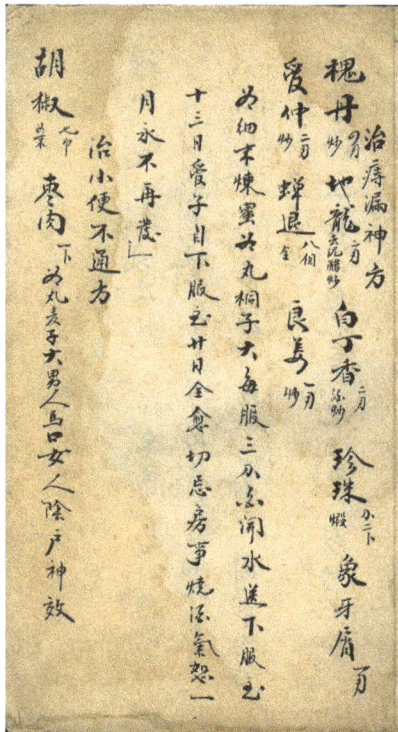

SURVEY OF CONTENTS: This is mainly a listing of 49 pharmaceutical recipes for the treatment of frequently encountered illnesses, such as piles, inability to pass urine, skin ailments and ulcers, pin-illness poisoning following the consumption of dead meat. The list includes fixed recipes with several components, as well as folk recipes with only one substance. Several pages of this volume deal with the pathological conditions of sand-illness, *sha zheng* 痧証. This section begins with a paragraph Sha yuan da lüe 痧原大略, "Broad outline of the origins of sand-illness". It outlines the major signs associated with the pathological condition of *sha* 痧, and then discusses numerous principles to be observed in the treatment of sand-illness conditions, *sha zheng* 痧証, such as Shao wu bu fa 痧無補法, "For sand-illness there is no method of supplementation," Yong yao da fa 用藥大法, "Major pattern of drug usage," Shi yin ji 食飲忌, "Taboos on solid food and beverages," Yao ji 藥忌, "Taboos on pharmaceutical substances" as well as a listing of numerous *sha* 痧 conditions and their recipes.

***

| | |
|---|---|
| TITLE: | (*Yi xue yuan li* 醫學原理, Medical principles) |
| ID: | 8857 |
| CONTENTS: | Medical theory |
| APPEARANCE: | Thin, simple manuscript volume. Exceptional calligraphy. Careful handwriting. Cover made of paper mulberry paper. No title. No table of contents. |
| BINDING: | Paper spills |
| MEASURE: | 16.7 x 12.7 |
| TITLE PAGE: | No. |
| NO. OF PAGES: | 13 |
| L.P. /CH.L: | 9 x 9-21 |
| LAYOUT: | No lines, no frames |
| AUTHOR AND YEAR OF TEXT: | |
| | Ming, Wang Ji 汪機, 1601 |
| YEAR OF COPY: | Character 弦 not written with a Qing-dynasty taboo observed. Republican era. |

SURVEY OF CONTENTS: This volume has two parts. The first 5 pages constitute the first part. The remaining pages are the second part. The first part has the title Nei jing shuo 內景說. It begins with Gong Yingyuan yun 龔應圓云

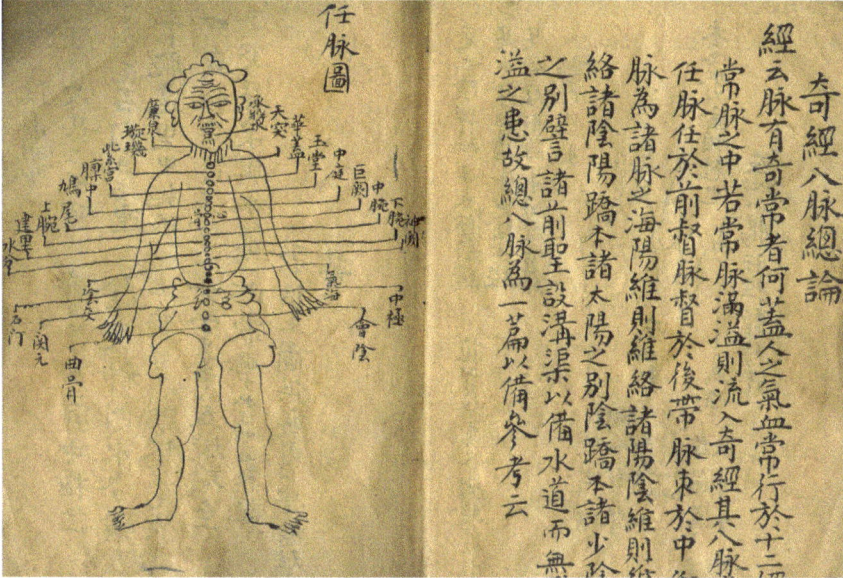

offering a systematic yet simple introduction to the human body's morpho-
logical sections. Gong Yingyuan 龔應圓 is Gong Juzong 龔居中, a famous late
Ming era physician from Jinxi 金溪 in Jiangxi 江西. Several of his writings do
still exist. From which of his books the section Nei jing shuo 內景說 was copied
remains to be examined.

The second part is a Qi jing ba mai zong lun 奇經八脈總論, copied from a
different book. Sections copied include 任脈圖、任脈歌、任脈圖論、任脈穴
二十有四、督脈圖、督脈歌、督脈圖論、督脈穴二十有七、衝脈論、帶脈
論、陽維脈論、陰維脈論、陽蹻脈論、陰蹻脈論.

A comparison shows that these contents were copied from the 2nd *juan* of
the Ming author Wang Ji's 汪機 *Yi xue yuan li* 醫學原理 of 1601. The *Yi xue yuan*
*li* 醫學原理 is extremely rare in China. It is surprising to see a folk manuscript
copy of this small medical-theoretical volume. The present text is a complete
copy of only the 2nd *juan*. Like *juan* 1 it includes drawings of and text on the
human body's conduit vessels.

***

TITLE:          *Yan ke. Xiao er tui na* 眼科·小兒推拿. Ophthalmology. Pedi-
                atric push-and-pull massage.
ID:             8858
CONTENTS:       Ophthalmology, Pediatrics

APPEARANCE: Ancient manuscript volume. Edges severely damaged. Paper color turned grey-yellow. No cover. Average calligraphy. Careful handwriting.

BINDING: Thread

MEASURE: 18.7 x 22.0

TITLE PAGE: No

NO. OF PAGES: 44

L.P. /CH.L: Ophthalmology part: 11 x 15

LAYOUT: No lines, no frames

AUTHOR AND YEAR OF TEXT:

Ming. Cheng Songya 程松崖. Copyist unknown.

YEAR OF COPY: The character 弦 is written without observing a Qing dynasty taboo. Republican era.

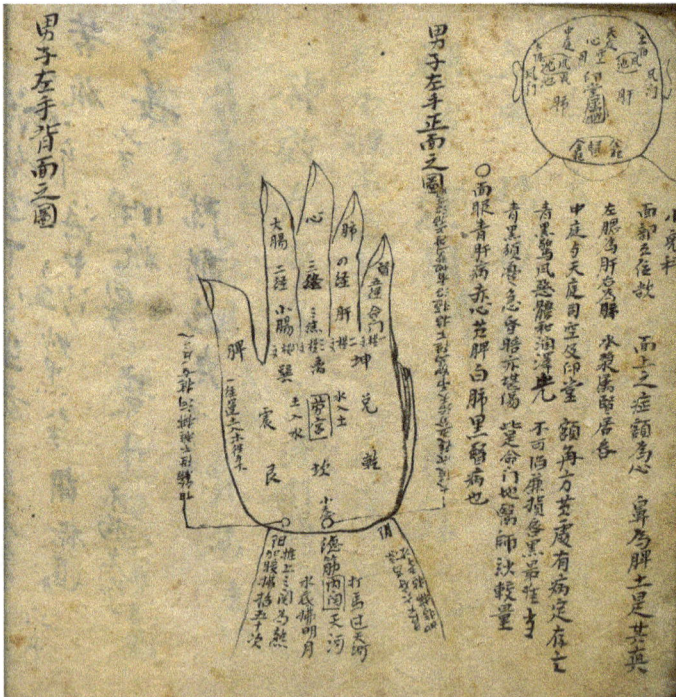

SURVEY OF CONTENTS: This volume combines diverse contents of medical texts. The first part is on ophthalmology; it begins with a drawing detailing the different sections of the eye. This is followed by a list of 17 eye afflictions, each illustrated by a separate drawing and followed by an explanatory text. Drawings and explanations match each other closely. Many of the drawings have

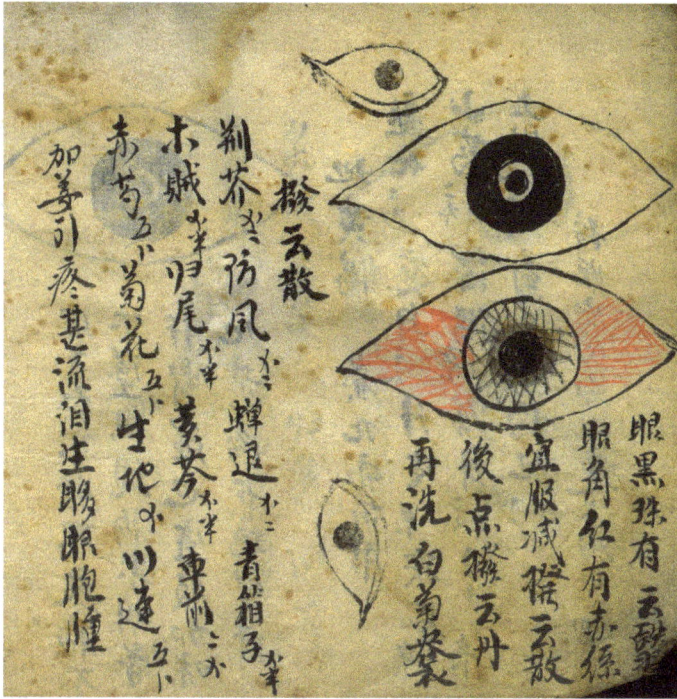

the affected section of the eye marked with red color – a very rare feature in such manuscript copies. A comparison shows that this part was copied from the Ming author Cheng Songya's 程松崖 *Yan ke ying yan liang fang* 眼科应验良方. It is followed by a listing of diverse pharmaceutical recipes, for example, "to treat tearflow without pain", *zhi yan liu lei bu teng* 治眼流淚不疼, and the "Elixir with *niu huang* and 8 valuable ingredients", *niu huang ba bao dan* 牛黄八寶丹.

A second part of the present volume has the title "Recipes transmitted by the old Mr. Zhu", Zhu lao xian sheng chuan fang 朱老先生傳方. Among the recipes listed are *bai ling wan* 百靈丸, *xiao ling dan* 小靈丹, and *jie gu dan* 接骨丹. Each recipe is accompanied by a careful explanation of the steps and methods of its preparation.

A third part is copied with small characters, obviously by a different person. The title is Xiao er ke, 小兒科, "Pediatrics". It begins with five drawings of, first, a child's face, a males's left palm, a male's back of the left hand, a female's palm of the right hand, and a female's back of the right hand. These drawing include numerous designations of locations on the face and the hands associated with the five long-term depots, the eight trigrams, etc. This is followed by four sections: Yang zhang tu ge xue shou fa xian jue 陽掌圖各穴手法仙訣, Yin zhang tu ge xue shou fa xian jue 陰掌圖各穴手法仙訣, San guan yao jue 三關要訣,

and Shou fa zhi bing jue 手法治病訣, the latter is a listing and explanation of 29 massage interventions.

A fourth part of this volume has the title Xiao er ke kan hu kou san guan 小兒科看虎口三關, "Pediatrics. Inspection of *hu kou* and *san guan*". It offers 20 drawings and explanations of a child's finger with characteristic lines used for diagnosis. This is followed by section Kan xiao er e yin tang shan gen 看小兒額印堂山根, "Inspection of a child's facial sections *yin tang* and *shan gen*". It offers data on a visual inspection of a child's facial sections designated as *yin tang* 印堂, *shan gen* 山根, *zheng kou* 正口, *cheng jiang liang mei* 承漿兩眉, *liang yan* 兩眼, *liang tai yang* 兩太陽 and *liang jian* 兩瞼.

Some of the contents of parts 3 and 4 described above are identical with those in ms. 8936. Perhaps they have originated in the same region. The *tuina* 推拿 push-and-pull massage is in the tradition of the Ming author Zhou Yufan's 周于藩 *Xiao er tui na mi jue* 小兒推拿秘訣.

A fifth part includes 57 diverse pharmaceutical recipes, mostly for therapies required in external medicine and traumatology. There is also a recipe for "fruits fried in oil", *chao you guo zi* 查（煠）油果子, i.e., an oil fried wheaten food.

The final two pages offer exorcistic therapies, including oral and written spells.

\*\*\*

| | |
|---|---|
| TITLE: | *Bai xing yi yao fang* 百姓醫藥方, Folk medical-pharmaceutical recipes. |
| ID: | 8859 |
| CONTENTS: | Pharmaceutical recipes |
| APPEARANCE: | Simple, ancient manuscript volume. Inferior calligraphy. Casual handwriting. Cover added later, with inscription in abbreviated characters by fountain pen: 百姓医药方. |
| BINDING: | Paper spills |
| MEASURE: | 21.9 x 11.0 |
| TITLE PAGE: | No |
| NO. OF PAGES: | 29 |
| L.P. /CH.L: | 8 x approx. 16 |
| LAYOUT: | No lines, no frames |
| AUTHOR AND YEAR OF TEXT: | |
| | Unknown |

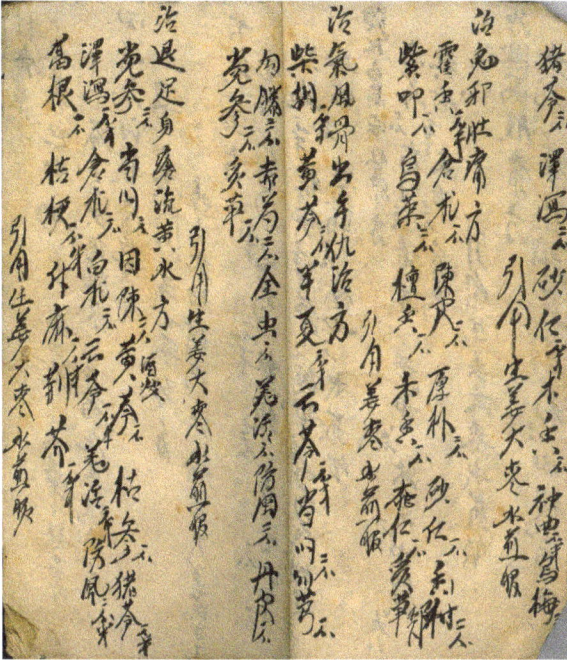

YEAR OF COPY: Paper quality and color of ink suggest that this volume was written in the Republican era.

SURVEY OF CONTENTS: This is a listing of more than 110 pharmaceutical recipes popular for treating commonly ᵉncountered ailments in the realms of gynecology, external medicine and internal medicine. These are mostly well-established recipes, such as *xiang sha yang wei tang* 香砂養胃湯 and *san zi yang qin tang* 三子養親湯. The volume also includes some rarely seen recipes.

\*\*\*

TITLE: (*Dan tai yu an. Mai zhen* 丹臺玉案·脈診, Cinnabar terrace and jade records. Vessel diagnosis)
ID: 8860
CONTENTS: Gynecology, Pulse diagnosis
APPEARANCE: Fine and well preserved ancient manuscript volume. Calligraphy above average. Characters of varying sizes. Cover made of paper mulberry paper. No title.
BINDING: Thread

MEASURE: 29.0 x 15.8
TITLE PAGE: No
NO. OF PAGES: 81
L.P. /CH.L: 6-12 x 25-32
LAYOUT: No lines, no frames
AUTHOR AND YEAR OF TEXT:
Ming. Sun Wenyin 孫文胤, 1637. Copyist unknown.
YEAR OF COPY: Paper quality and absence of characters written to observe Qing dynasty taboos suggest that this volume was written in the Republican era.

SURVEY OF CONTENTS: The contents of this volume are clearly summarized in a line of eight characters on the back of the first page: 婦科、雜抄、偏方、脈理. The volume is not introduced by a title on the cover, but an identification is possible nevertheless. From page 1 through p. 13, a listing of pharmaceutical recipes is presented, mostly with very few ingredients or constituting of a single substance so that they are easy to use. Beginning with p. 14 a second part of this volume has the title *Nü ke. Dan tai yü an* 女科，丹台玉案. A comparison shows that this section is a complete copy of *juan* 5, Fu ren ke婦人科, of the Ming author Sun Wenyin's 孫文胤 *Dan tai yü an* 丹臺玉案 of 1637. At the end of this section, the copyist added the following note: 丹臺玉案一書，系予在原平時從恒德有借一爛本照抄，故不知何代書，亦不知何謂丹臺玉案也。所抄有方有病門而無方藥歌訣。予將方後糊編歌訣。倘後人有學是道者，使之誦二易記也。予又將幾宗藥治何病為要者，亦糊編之，抄後亦待記之，以備臨時易於擇用也. That is, some of the contents were not copied from the *Dan tai yü an*, but were added by the copyist himself.

The section copied from the *Dan tai yü an* is followed by a poem rhymed in four characters per line on vessel diagnosis, with commentaries. The volume concludes with rhymed instructions on pharmaceutical recipes.

***

TITLE:              *You ke tui na shu chao ji* 幼科推拿書抄輯, Manuscript edition of a text on pediatric push-and-pull-massage.

ID:                 8861

CONTENTS:           Pediatrics

APPEARANCE:         Exquisite ancient manuscript volume with edges slightly damaged. Small characters beautifully written with above average calligraphy. Cover made of paper mulberry paper. No title given.

BINDING:            Thread

MEASURE:            18.0 x 14.0

TITLE PAGE:         Two. Second with inscription: 推拿書.

NO. OF PAGES:       76

L.P. /CH.L:         8 x 19

LAYOUT:             No lines, no frames

AUTHOR AND YEAR OF TEXT:
                    Qing. Luo Rulong 駱如龍, 1725

YEAR OF COPY:       No Qing dynasty taboos on 搐 and 弦 observed. Republican era.

SURVEY OF CONTENTS: In the paragraph Xue dao lun 穴道論, a quote is introduced as *Qian'an yue* 潛庵曰, "Qian'an states". Qian'an is the alternative name of the Qing physician and author Luo Rulong 駱如龍. A comparison shows that most of the contents of this volume was copied from his *You ke tui na bi shu* 幼科推拿秘書. The sequence of chapters in the present volume mostly follows that of the original book. However, its contents are much broader than those of Luo Rulong's text. For example, the Zong lun 總論, "Summary", at the beginning of the present volume was copied from the Qing author Xiong

Yingxiong's 熊應雄 *Xiao er tui na kuang yi* 小兒推拿廣意 of 1676. We have not been able to search for the origins of all paragraphs added to Luo Rulong's book in the present volume. It may be concluded, though, that Lu Rulong's book constitutes the basis of the present volume, with apparent additions copied from further source texts.

***

| | |
|---|---|
| TITLE: | *Huang Di nei jing ling shu zhu zheng fa wei* 黃帝內經靈樞註證發微, A commentary elucidating the *Huang Di nei jing ling shu* |
| ID: | 8862 |
| CONTENTS: | Medical classic |
| APPEARANCE: | Ancient manuscript with new dark blue cover made from tough paper prepared from bast fibre of the paper mulberry. Calligraphy above average. Handwriting careful. No title. |
| BINDING: | Thread, new |

MEASURE:              20.5 x 13.2

TITLE PAGE:           Vertical title on the left: 霛樞內經卷二上，on the right: 經
                      脈十上

NO. OF PAGES:         61

L.P. /CH.L:           10 x. 21

LAYOUT:               No lines, no frames

AUTHOR AND YEAR OF TEXT:

                      Ming, Ma Shi 馬蒔, Yuan tai 元臺.

YEAR OF COPY:         Paper quality and absence of characters written to observe
                      Qing dynasty taboos suggest that this volume was written in
                      the Republican era.

SURVEY OF CONTENTS: This is a handwritten copy of the Ming author Ma
Shi's printed book *Huang Di nei jing ling shu zhu zheng fa wei* 黃帝內經靈樞註
證發微 – a very famous commentated version of the *Ling shu* 靈樞 in 9 *juan*
from the end of the Ming dynasty. However, the present volume is fragmentary
as it includes only *juan* 2, discussing the chapter Jing mai, di shi 經脈第十,
"Conduit vessels, no. 10", of the original *Ling shu*. The items treated include the
long-term depots, short-term repositories, and conduits, and are illustrated by
numerous drawings of organs and conduits.

***

TITLE:                *Kun lun shan zong jue* 崑崙山總訣, Comprehensive instruc-
                      tions from Kunlun mountain

ID:                   8863

CONTENTS:             Geomancy

APPEARANCE:           Two ancient manuscript volumes. Good quality. Above av-
                      erage calligraphy. Cover made from common cotton paper.
                      The 1st volume with an inscription from left to right: 崑崙山
                      總訣上冊　不借出門，免開尊口緊記/江隆煌備用/民國拾
                      叁年歲次甲子孟冬月抄錄. The 2nd volume has an identi-
                      cal inscription, except for stating 下冊, instead of 上冊. No
                      table of contents.

BINDING:              Thread

MEASURE:              23.0 x 12.7

TITLE PAGE:           No

NO. OF PAGES:      Vol. 1: 51, vol. 2: 52

L.P. /CH.L:        10 x approx. 24

LAYOUT:         No lines, no frames

AUTHOR AND YEAR OF TEXT:    Unknown

YEAR OF COPY:   Character 玄 written to observe a Qing dynasty taboo. Nevertheless, the cover states: 1925.

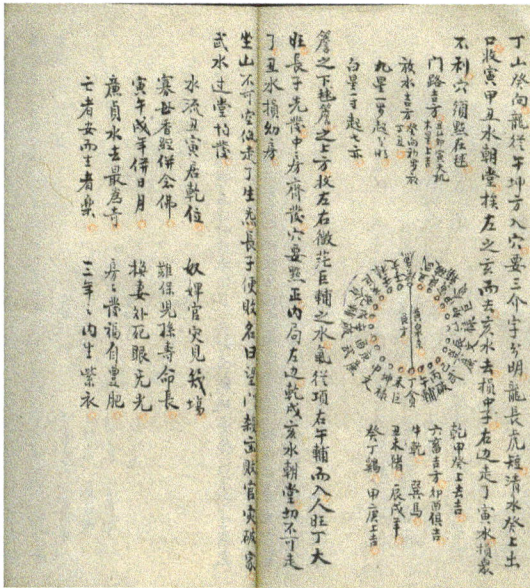

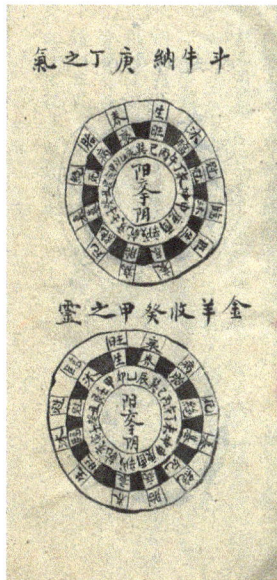

SURVEY OF CONTENTS: This is a book on *kan yu* 堪輿, another term for *feng shui* 風水, i.e., geomancy. Its focus is on theory, including Yin-Yang 陰陽- and Five Phases 五行-doctrines, with discourses on mountains, waters, homes, and tombs. The text discusses difficult issues, such as where to open water ditches, *shui lu* 水路, where to place a door, *men lu* 門路, mountain directions, et al. The contents are not immediately related to diagnosis and therapy in medicine.

*** 

| | |
|---|---|
| TITLE: | (*Kan yu yao zhi* 堪輿要旨, Essentials of geomancy ) |
| ID: | 8864 |
| CONTENTS: | Geomancy, Feng shui |
| APPEARANCE: | Ancient manuscript volume. Average calligraphy. Disorderly handwriting. Cover made from kraft paper. No title. Several empty pages prior to the beginning of the main text. |
| BINDING: | Original threads lost. Replaced by more recent metal staples. |
| MEASURE: | 21 x 14.6 |
| TITLE PAGE: | No |
| NO. OF PAGES: | 56 |
| L.P. /CH.L: | 8 – 10 x >24 |
| LAYOUT: | No lines, no frames |

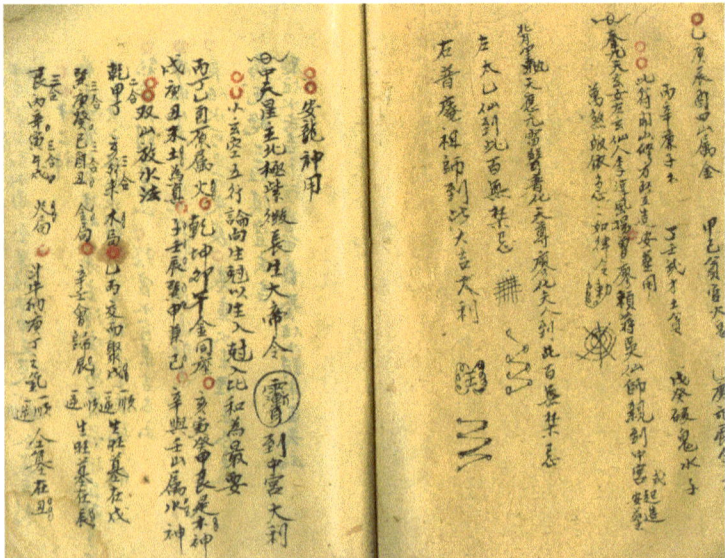

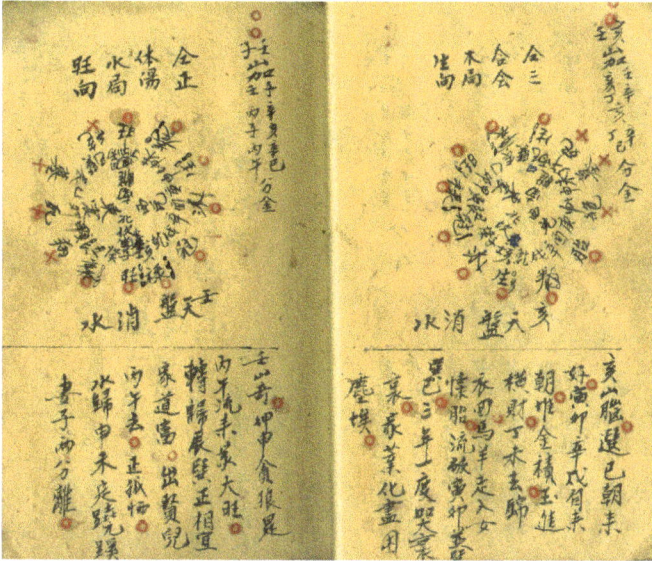

**AUTHOR AND YEAR OF TEXT:**
Unknown

YEAR OF COPY: Character 玄 not written to observe a Qing dynasty taboo. Republican era.

SURVEY OF CONTENTS: This volume focusses on *kan yu* 堪輿, i.e., *feng shui* 風水, geomancy. The paragraph Yao zhi 要旨, "Essentials", states: 入山觀水口，登穴看明堂氣。欲識真龍行與居，且看水局來與去. The text is not directly related to diagnosis and treatment in medicine.

\*\*\*

TITLE: (*Shi yong za fang ben* 使用雜方本, Miscellaneous recipes for practical use）

ID: 8865

CONTENTS: Pharmaceutical recipes

APPEARANCE: Ancient manuscript volume. Cover made of common cotton paper. Slightly damaged. Edges folded. Inscription: 使用雜貨本/李生發記. Average calligraphy.

BINDING: Thread.

MEASURE: 29.3 x 14.0

TITLE PAGE: No

NO. OF PAGES: 31

L.P. /CH.L: 6 – 7 x approx. 26

LAYOUT: No lines, no frames

AUTHOR AND YEAR OF TEXT:

Unknown, Copyist: Li Shengfa 李生發.

YEAR OF COPY: No Qing dynasty taboos observed. Paper quality and nature of ink suggest that this volume was written during the Republican era.

SURVEY OF CONTENTS: The title on the cover says "Volume for useful sundry goods", *Shi yong za huo ben* 使用雜貨本. However, no sundry goods whatsoever are recorded. Presumably, this volume was meant to be used for recording sundry goods, but was then converted to a collection of pharmaceutical recipes. Hence we have given it the title *Shi yong za fang ben* 使用雜方本, "Volume for useful pharmaceutical recipes." In all, 168 recipes are listed. Their sequence follows no apparent order; they are not categorized in any way. They include some established recipes with several ingredients, in addition to many small recipes with only very few ingredients. Most indications are from the realm of gynecology and, to a lesser amount, external medicine. Apparently, this is a collection of recipes popular among the general population.

***

TITLE: (*Fu zhou hui ji* 符咒汇集, Collected charms and spells)
ID: 8866
CONTENTS: Exorcism
APPEARANCE: Ancient manuscript. Cover damaged. No title. Paper brittle. Each page with printed red producer information: 佛鎮高盛造. Handwriting with small characters. Calligraphy above average.

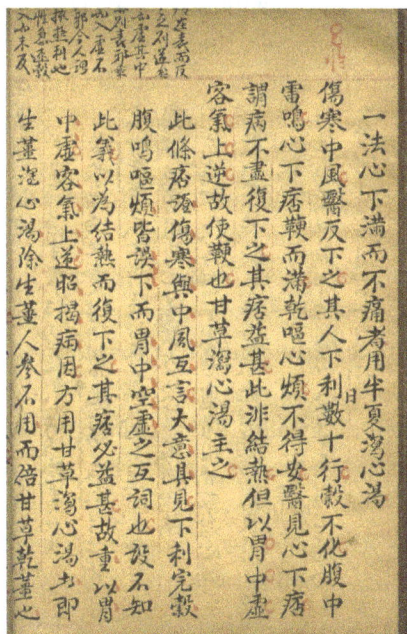

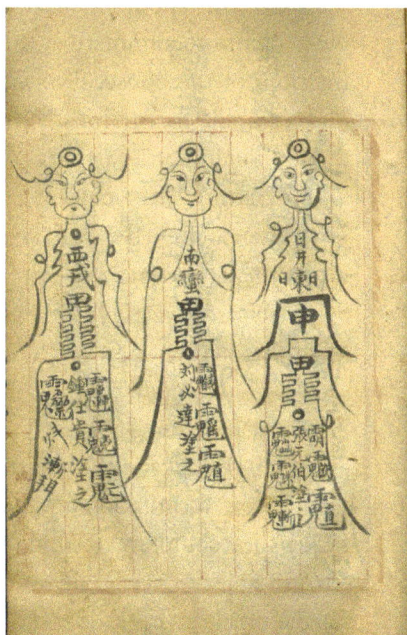

BINDING: Thread
MEASURE: 19.6 x 14.0
TITLE PAGE: No
NO. OF PAGES: 75

L.P. /CH.L:          10 – 15 x approx. 19, with many charms interspersed in the
                     text.

LAYOUT:              10 red lines; red frames. Two broad margins above and be-
                     low.

AUTHOR AND YEAR OF TEXT:
                     Unknown

YEAR OF COPY:        Character 玄 written to observe taboo with last stroke omit-
                     ted. End of Qing dynasty.


SURVEY OF CONTENTS: This is a manuscript record of exorcistic texts and
charms. Among the latter are many drawn in forms not seen elsewhere. The
contents of this volume are mainly as follows, listed here following their sequence in the volume.

1.      "Incantation to remove what is unclean", Qu hui zhou 去穢咒. Including
        phrases to be avoided and four charm-type charms.

2.      ("Thunder command" type charms – these titles of sections worded by
        ZJS/PUU. This applies to all titles of sections mentioned in brackets be-
        low). Charm to eliminate evil. Charm to suppress the queer. Charm for
        the door of the house. Five thunders charm, etc., together 30 charms.
        These graphic charms mostly carry a "thunder command", lei ling 雷令, at
        the top. Such charms are rarely seen elsewhere.

3.      (Tai ji charm) These charms are mostly not designed to suppress evil.
        They often address the stars, such as the "five stars of the polar star in the
        East", dong dou wu xing 東斗五星 and the "six stars of the polar star in the
        South", nan dou liu xing 南斗六星. There is also an "amulet to protect the
        altar", hu tan fu 護壇符, and a "seal of the mysterious girl", xuan nü yin shi
        玄女印式, written in red.

4.      "The true man Sun [Simiao's] method of needling the 13 demon holes",
        Sun zhen ren shi san gui xue zhen fa 孫真人十三鬼穴針法. This section
        includes an "Incantation to catch the evil", Zhao xie zhou 罩邪咒; "Incan-
        tation to accompany needling patterns", Zhou zhen fa zhou 咒針法咒;
        "The 13 holes to needle demons", Shi san zhen gui xue 十三針鬼穴; "To
        needle diseases [caused by the] evil", Zhen xie bing 針邪病; "The minor
        celestial gang star incantation", Xiao tian gang zhou 小天罡咒, as well
        as "Taboos prohibiting needling and cauterization because of the pres-
        ence of the human spirit", Zhen jiu ren shen jin ji 鍼灸人神禁忌, "Hours
        and days suitable for needling and cauterizing", Zhen jiu shi ri 鍼灸時日.
        There is also a list of 28 insertion holes. This section falls into the realm

of acupuncture and moxibustion. It ends with a paragraph Yin yang ba zhang 陰陽把掌, informing of a therapy method by means of blowing qi and clasping the hands.

5. (Amulet modules) These are very small charms. They appear like modules used to generate larger charms. Examples are: 川真符、請仙符、天尊符、送仙符、翰真人、童子符、請戰仙法, etc.

6. Pharmaceutical recipes: Recipes to drain, *xie fang* 瀉方; Recipes to make someone fall to the ground, *dao fang* 倒方; Medication to implant a disease, *zhong bing fang* 種病藥 (with ingredients: *shan bi ma* 山蓖麻, *ma qian zi* 馬前子, *chan su* 蟬酥); Recipes to dissolve, *jie fang* 解方, Recipe for knock-out medication, *meng yao fang* 蒙藥方, "take *cao wu* 草烏, *qing fen* 輕粉 plus *ren yan* 人言 [i.e., *xin shi* 信石], *jin tou wu gong mao wei* 金頭蜈蚣毛尾, complete, *ban mao* 班毛, and *chan su* 蟬酥. Prepare a fine powder. Paste on the forehead with *nan xing* 南星. [The person thus manipulated will] shout *ai* and fall to the ground;" Recipe for malaria, *nue ji fang* 瘧疾方; "[Recipe to] eliminate mosqitoes", *wu wen* 無蚊; "[Recipe to eliminate] stinking bugs", *chou chong* 臭蟲, etc.

7. *Guang fa* 光法: meaning unclear.

8. Worship, *ji* 祭; interdictions, *jin* 禁; incantations, *zhou* 咒: *ji bi zhou* 祭筆咒, "incantation far sacrifices by means of a pen"; *ji mo zhou* 祭墨咒, "incantation for sacrifices by means of ink"; *jin fang huo zhou* 禁防火咒, "incantation to disallow fire"; *feng wan zhou* 封碗咒, "incantation to seal a bowl"; *jiu huo fu* 救火符, "amulet to save from fire".

9. Patterns to arrest a thief with the aid of the eight trigrams, Ba gua ding zei fa 八卦定賊法: 治賊法、賊盜喪膽法; Amulet for all doors (These are doors towards the different cardinal directions), *ge men fu* 各門符; "Amulet for disharmony", *bu he fu* 不和符, "Amulet to hold down the white tiger", *zhen bai hu fu* 鎮白虎符; "Amulet to protect the body", *hu shen fu* 護身符; ["Amulet ] to hold down the scarlet bird", *zhen zhu qiao* 鎮朱雀, "Planet Jupiter charm", *sui xing fu* 歲星符

10. "Divine incantation to cure disease and eliminate evil on imperial command paper", Zhi bing qu xie chi zhi shen zhou 治病驅邪敕紙神咒: to command water, inkstone, ink, and pen, to direct a request to the gods, to clean the altar: 敕水、硯、墨、筆、請神、淨壇......

11. *Yang lei fa shu* 陽雷法術; *hu li yu bao* 狐狸預報; *zhui hun suo ren fu* 追魂鎖人符; *wu lei shen shou fa* 五雷神手法

12. "Secret oral instructions and charms to dispel evil", 除邪符式口訣: 外天罡、召天罡、安壇咒、淨壇咒、淨心咒、淨口咒、淨身咒、淨天地

咒、斬仙劍、總符、內天罡、外天罡...... At the end are 斬邪符、拘邪符、追赴符、請神符、除邪符、拿精符、斬鬼符、護身符、上枷符、上扭符、收禁符、八王符諱 (a charm in the shape of a human head)、覆地符、滴血咒、催神咒、起霧咒、運筆符、遣邪符 (many different charms)、保命符、除邪符、霹靂、(many seal-type charms)、陽鎖符、簿箕符、都土地符、玉皇符、韋陀符、三臺符、吞符化百邪 (in the shape of a centipede)、王翁符。

13. Gesture patterns: a collection of more than 90 manual gestures, *shou jue* 手訣, and manual prints, *shou yin* 手印, followed by 68 illustrations.

14. Secret instructions for facing evil, *xiang xie mi jue* 相邪秘訣：解法、治法、斬邪法、捉邪法、奪邪法、熏邪法、鎖邪法、拘邪法、赴身咒、罩邪咒、運氣咒、三十八宿咒 (with graphic charms added）

To conclude: The various types of charms appear not connected, and a systematic sequence is not obvious. However, because of its diversity and rich contents this manuscript volume is certainly worth further attention.

***

TITLE:          *Zhong hua xin zhen jiu* 中華新鍼灸, New acupuncture of China

ID:             8867

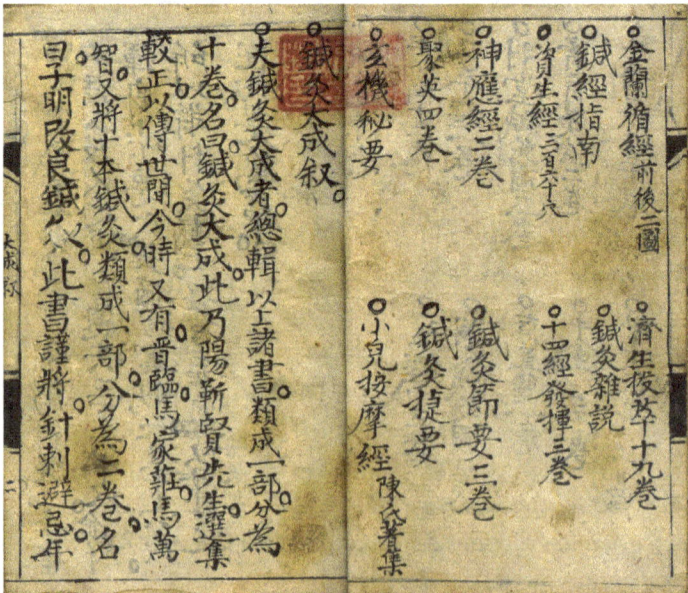

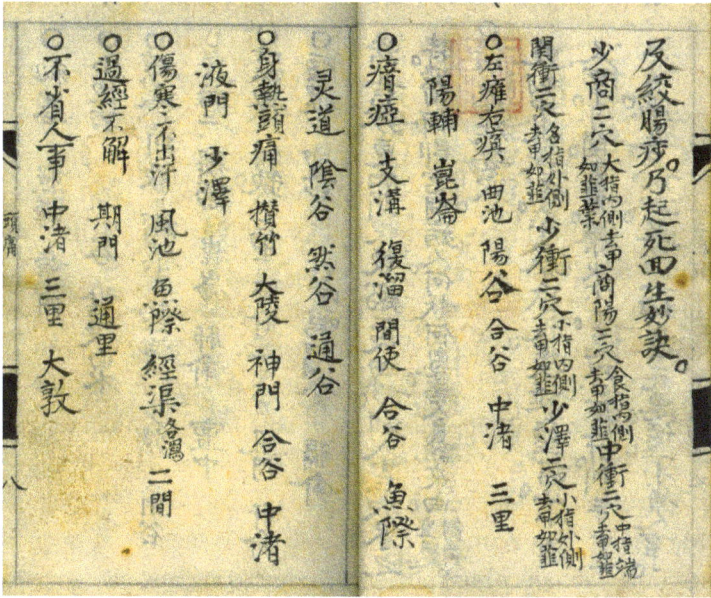

| CONTENTS: | Acupuncture |
|---|---|
| APPEARANCE: | Ancient manuscript volume in cardboard case with blue fabric exterior. External front with paper label. Handwritten title: 中華新鍼灸. Two vols. with sturdy cover each, made from several layers of paper glued to each other. Careful handwriting. Average calligraphy. Front page with inscription: 子明改良鍼灸/擇之/晋臨馬家莊/名馬萬智/字馬子明. |
| BINDING: | Thread |
| MEASURE: | 16.8 x 11.4 |
| TITLE PAGE: | 1st vol. with inscription: 中華新鍼灸/晋臨/馬子明編. |
| NO. OF PAGES: | Vol. 1: 83 (of these 65 pp. 中華新鍼灸); vol. 2: 69 (of these 62 pp. 中華新鍼灸). Edges with black fish tale in upper half. |
| L.P. /CH.L: | 6 x approx. 24 |
| LAYOUT: | Single line frame on all four sides of the text. No lines between columns of characters. |

AUTHOR AND YEAR OF TEXT:

Republican era, Ma Wanzhi 馬萬智, Ziming 子明.

YEAR OF COPY: Republican era.

SURVEY OF CONTENTS: This book was authored by a folk physician named Ma Wanzhi 馬萬智, Ziming 子明, of Shanxi 山西 province. The two handwritten volumes are designed to copy the appearance of printed books. The cover has a label with the title; the text is preceded by a preface. The main text is surrounded by a rectangular line frame. However, the *Zhong guo zhong yi yao gu ji mu lu* 中國中醫古籍總目 does not list this book. Also an author-physician named Ma Wanzhi does not appear in any other bibliographical work. Hence this may have been a privately produced and only personally used book on acupuncture.

The text in vol. 1 is not homogenous. In its preface, Zhen jiu da cheng xu 鍼灸大成敘, the author states: "Now, the *Zhen jiu da cheng* was compiled by using all types of previous texts. Their contents were rearranged and divided into ten *juan* with the title *Zhen jiu da cheng* 鍼灸大成. This then was a compilation by Mr. Yang 陽 [i.e., Yang Jizhou 楊繼洲], and it was re-edited by Mr. Jin Xian 靳賢, to be transmitted to the world. Recently, in Jinlin 晋臨, in the village of the Ma family, Ma jia zhuang 馬家莊, Mr. Ma Wanzhi 馬萬智 once again rearranged the contents of ten books on acupuncture and cauterization into one book, divided into 2 *juan*, and gave it the title *Zi ming gai liang zhen jiu* 子明改良鍼灸, "Acupuncture and cauterization improved by Ziming". This book carefully relates taboos to be observed when piercing with needles, as well as years, months, days and hours. It includes all of that. In addition it includes five sections on needle incantations for supplementation and drainage, patterns of how to select the insertion opening, and it also covers all 360 insertion holes spread all over the human body. In my [text here] I have selected 216 insertion holes from head to toe as most important. Hence it covers the most essential statements and insertion holes for acupuncture and cauterization therapy."

Apparently, the author's level of education was not very high. His book was written as a digest of the *Zhen jiu da cheng* 鍼灸大成. The author excerpted passages to explain the locations of needle insertion holes, and the depth of an appropriate insertion, as well as the number of moxibustion cones to be burned at a location. He also provided brief statements on therapeutic effects to be achieved by treating at each insertion/cauterization point.

Vol. 2 is different. The sequence of sections is as follows: 背穴要歌, 井荥俞原经合歌, 馬丹陽天星十二穴治雜病歌, 四總穴歌, 玉龍歌, 回陽九針歌, 孫真人十三鬼穴, and 治急症要穴. All these sections are on acupuncture. They are followed by two sections "Pediatrics", Xiao er ke 小兒科, and "Males, females, old, young," Nan nü lao you 男女老幼, listing numerous illnesses to be treated with acupuncture, push-and-pull massage (*tui na* 推拿) and pharmaceutical recipes. The volume concludes with long lists of pharmaceutical recipes.

This book is the outcome of a rural healer's intention to write a book. It offers neither new ideas nor follows a noteworthy style and structure.

On the inside of the covers the two volumes have notes written on pharmaceutical recipes, including exorcistic approaches, as well as riddles concerning insertion points and pharmaceutical substances. They appear unrelated to the main contents of this book.

***

TITLE:            (*Tie da xue shang* 跌打穴傷, Harm received at insertion
                  holes by falls and blows)
ID:               8868
CONTENTS:         Bone setting – Traumatology
APPEARANCE:       Ancient manuscript volume with an exquisite cover, in a
                  brand-new case in blue cloth. A small paper label is glued to
                  the outside with an inscription: 跌打穴傷 (全圖一冊). Main
                  text: average calligraphy. Drawings inferior.

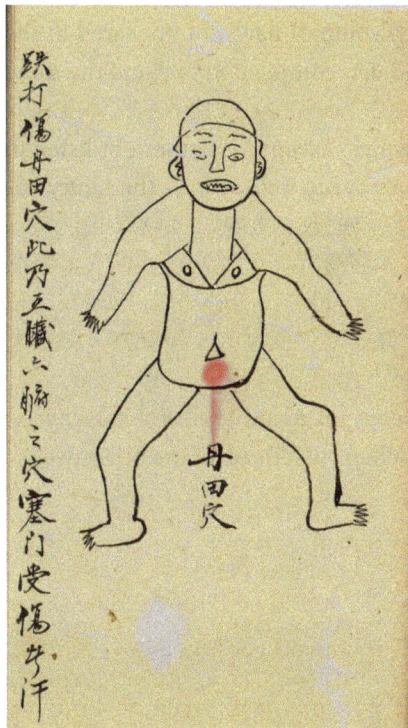

BINDING:          Beautifully bound with gold-color thread
MEASURE:          26,0 x 15,4
TITLE PAGE:       No
NO. OF PAGES:     26
L.P. /CH.L:       Pages without drawings: 7-8 x approx. 21
LAYOUT:           No lines, no frames
AUTHOR AND YEAR OF TEXT:
                  Anonymous. Qing dynasty. Copyist unknown.
YEAR OF COPY:     Character 玄 is written with the final stroke omitted. End of
                  Qing dynasty.

SURVEY OF CONTENTS: This volumes offers knowledge of folk healers of former times to treat illnesses associated with bone setting and traumatology.
Such writings were widely distributed among the people. They focus on injuries and insertion holes for treatment. Closely related to the current volume
are vols. 8845 and 8852. Their common characteristic are drawings of the human body showing the location (and its name) where an injury was received
and naming the pharmaceutical substances to be resorted to for therapy. The
volumes agree in the naming of many of the locations and hence may have
originated from an identical source. Such volumes have not appeared in the
Berlin collections before. They may have been compiled in one and the same
region.

In all, the present volume has 26 drawings. Except for names not listed in
the two other volumes, the names refer always to holes where the injury has
taken place. They include the following: 嬌空穴、太陽穴·太陰穴·囟門穴、
咽喉正穴、血腕下穴、乳膀穴、乃膀穴、將臺穴、牙腮穴、心頭穴、雙燕
入洞穴、（肚）臍穴、童子骨穴、下竅穴、丹田穴、下陰穴、田池穴、背
梁骨穴、對口穴、同（銅）壺滴漏穴、鳳轉穴、鳳尾穴、掛膀穴、腰上大
穴、人宮穴。

To treat injured "holes" this volume relies on pharmaceutical substances.
The contents of this volume are even sketchier than those of the other two.

***

TITLE:            *Ji yan liang fang* 集驗良方, Proven, good recipes
ID:               8869
CONTENTS:         Pharmaceutical recipes

APPEARANCE:    Eight ancient manuscript volumes of identical size and cover of an original set of 9 volumes. Nice with distinct handwriting., and calligraphy above average. Volumes 1, 2, 3, and 9 designated on front cover below the title with vol. 1, 2, 3, etc. The remaining three have no such obvious identification, neither outside nor inside. One volume consists of two parts. A first part is a printed text on tongue diagnosis. The second, much larger part is a handwritten text on pulse diagnosis.

BINDING:    Thread

MEASURE:    17.0 x 12.2

TITLE PAGE:    Handwritten vols.: No. 1 vol. with printed text: see below

NO. OF PAGES:    Vol. 1: 45. Vol. 2: 53. Vol. 3: 38. Vol. 4: 42. Vol. 5: 49. Vol. 6: 45. Vol. 7: 44. Vol. 8: 16 printed; 37 handwritten.

L.P. /CH.L:    Uneven. Mostly 7 x 16.

LAYOUT:    No lines, no frames. Exception: printed pages bound together with handwritten text.

AUTHOR AND YEAR OF TEXT:

    Uneven. Vol. 1 with date *tong zhi* 同治 reign period, 3rd year, i.e., 1864.

YEAR OF COPY:    In most of the volumes, the character 玄 was not written to observe a Qing dynasty taboo.

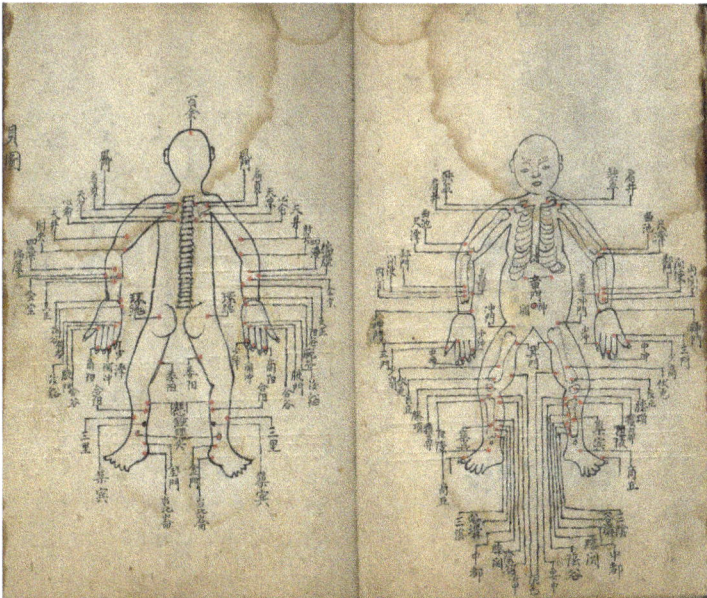

SURVEY OF CONTENTS: Vol. 1 has a short preface signed with a date 同治三年
正月, "*tong zhi* reign period, 3rd year, 1st month" (1864), but not with the name
of an author. This preface does not go into any detail and provides no hints
at the book's origin and contents. The preface is followed by four drawings of
human bodies with designations of body parts and needle insertion holes. The

subsequent text has the following sections: 經絡臟腑相配、脈訣應用、藥十八反歌、妊娠服藥禁用歌、腫瘍類方目錄 (an introduction to 25 recipes, plus 2 further attached recipes), 潰瘍主治目錄 (an introduction to 26 recipes, plus 1 ophthalmological recipe), and 腫瘍敷貼論. Seen together the contents of this volume are rather diverse, lacking a special focus.

Vol. 2 begins with a table of contents providing simple key terms informing one of the nature and indications of the recipes listed subsequently. The key terms are the following: ["medication] to cleanse", *xi tiao* 洗滌; ointment medication, *gao yao* 膏藥; "powder to stabilize pain", *ding tong san* 定痛散; medication for anesthesia, *ma yao* 麻藥; "divine lamp [wick] cauterization", *shen deng zhao* 神燈照; "interdiction of sores", *jin chuang* 禁瘡; "eye section", *mu bu* 目部; "head section", *tou bu* 頭部; "tooth section", *chi bu* 齒部; "ear section", *er bu* 耳部; "mouth section", *kou bu* 口部; "throat section", *hou bu* 喉部; "blood spitting", *tu xue* 吐血; "nosebleed", *bi xue* 鼻血; "powder to open the joints", *kai guan san* 開關散; "hand section", *shou bu* 手部; "scrophula", *luo li* 瘰癧; "breast section", *ru bu* 乳部; "gullet occlusion", *ye ge* 噎嗝; "drum [belly] distension", *gu zhang* 鼓腫 (appendix: *gu* swelling, *gu zhang* 蟲脹; "accumulation swelling", *ji zhang* 積脹); "lesion from sitting on a latrine board", *zuo ban chuang* 坐板瘡; "pemphigus", *tian pao chuang* 天皰瘡. The recipes are listed with most sections introduced by headings of a different structure, some repeating only the key terms from the table of contents, others adding the two characters 类方, for example 洗滌类方, "recipes to cleanse". In all, this volume lists more than 120 recipes. It also includes an exorcistic section Jin chuang ke fa 禁瘡科法, "Method from the specialty of banning ulcers," suggesting 12 different exorcistic characters for each month of a year to be written down accompanied by verbal spells to exorcise demons responsible for an ulcer. A section Shen deng zhao fa 神燈照法 outlines various approaches of lamp wick cauterization, a folk therapy.

Vol. 3, again, begins with a table of 21 key terms, such as *fu tong* 腹痛, "abdominal pain", *ke sou* 咳嗽, "cough", to introduce 123 recipes listed subsequently. The headings of the 21 sections simply repeat these key terms; the structure xx類方 is not repeated here. Often following a heading several pages have remained blank. Apparently, the autor of this volume intended to record recipes for certain therapeutic indications at some later time.

Vol. 4 begins with a table of contents added by a later hand, listing more than 30 therapeutic illnesses from the realm of external medicine and introducing a total of 125 recipes.

Vol. 5 begins with a table of contents listing 41 therapeutic indications from the realms of internal medicine, particular body parts, such as *er zheng* 耳症,

"ear conditions", *bi bu* 鼻部, "nose section", *kou she* 口舌, "mouth and tongue", as well as from gynecology and external medicine, introducing a total of 96 recipes.

Vol. 6 is entirely devoted to pediatric smallpox. Its table of contents lists 29 sections beginning with general discourses, such as Ren dou zhi fa 認痘之法, "Patterns to assess smallpox," Dou you wu ban 痘有五般, "There are five types of smallpox," Dou chuang zhi fa 痘瘡治法, "Therapy patterns for smallpox ulcers", and ending with specific pathological conditions associated with smallpox, such as *han zhan* 寒戰, "shivering", *yao ya* 咬牙, "grinding of the teeth", *niao se* 尿澀, "urine roughness", and *bian bi* 便秘, "constipation". The text suggests more than 60 recipes for treatment.

Vol. 7 is devoted to applications of the "fire needle", i.e., moxibustion with a mugwort stick, *huo zhen jiu* 火針灸. The volume includes 22 drawings of the human body showing the locations of two or more needle insertion holes that can also be used for moxibustion. Each drawing is accompanied by text explaining the use and therapeutic indications associated with each location. The volume's final pages were written by a different hand. They deal with smallpox and seem to have been added here erroneously rather than to vol. 6 where they belong.

Vol. 9 has a first section that is a printed text, and a second section that is handwritten. The printed text has the title *Chong ke shang han shi yan jing fa san she liu she tu* 重刊傷寒世驗精法三十六舌圖. It was published by Wu Xiaoting 吳孝亭 from Guan zhong 關中 in the first year of the *tong zhi* 同治 reign period (1862). The author is identified on the first page as 河東古芮春臺張吾仁纂. This book was widely disseminated. The subsequent handwritten part begins with a discourse "On the main conduits and network vessels where in case of harm caused by cold the disease is received", Shang han shou bing jing luo lun 傷寒受病經絡論, followed by seven pharmaceutical recipes. They are followed by a Mai fu 脈賦, "Poem on the movement in the vessels", and subsequent paragraphs bearing the titles: 診脈入式歌、診婦人有妊歌、七表脈歌、八里脈歌, 九道脈歌, and so on. They all were copied from the *Wang Shuhe mai jue* 王叔和脈訣. The handwriting of this volume differs from that in the other volumes. The character 玄 was written to observe a Qing dynasty taboo.

\*\*\*

TITLE:              *Yao xing fu zhi zhang* 藥性賦指掌, A guide to the *Yao xing fu*.
ID:                 8870
CONTENTS:           Materia medica

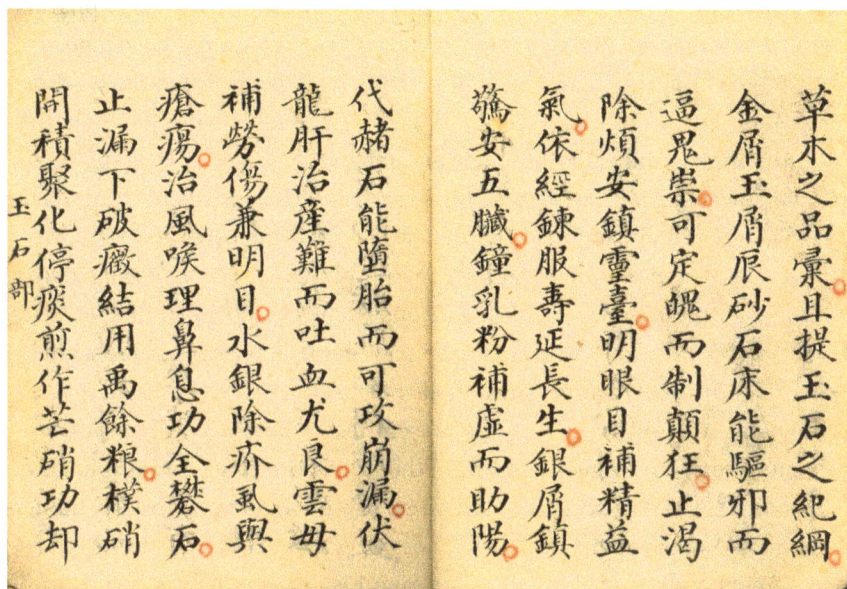

APPEARANCE:         Small, pocket-size ancient manuscript volume. Excellent
                    calligraphy. Careful handwriting. Front cover with inscrip-
                    tion: 藥性賦指掌/醫林書室藏本. Back of title page with in-
                    scription: 是賦也，其詞磊落，其文簡便，令人無望洋浩
                    歎之苦，輔醫道有易記誦之功，是以為序。後學竹溪氏
                    識，思聖

BINDING:            Thread
MEASURE:            14.2 x 11.9
TITLE PAGE:         Yes, with inscription: 藥性賦指掌/光緒二十二年晚秋立/道
                    生堂記
NO. OF PAGES:       32
L.P. /CH.L:         6 x 12
LAYOUT:             No lines, no frames
AUTHOR AND YEAR OF TEXT:
                    Ming, Luo Biwei 羅必煒, Copied by Dao sheng tang 道生堂.

YEAR OF COPY:     The title page states *guang xu* 光緒 reign period, 22nd year,
                  i.e., 1896. However, in the main text the character 玄 was
                  not written to observe a Qing dynasty taboo. Hence this text
                  may have been copied in the Republican era.

SURVEY OF CONTENTS: This is a "rhymed account of the nature of pharmaceutical substances", *Yao xing fu* 藥性賦. The title *Yao xing fu zhi zhang* 藥性
賦指掌 written on the cover and on the title page is not listed in the *Zhong
guo zhong yi gu ji zong mu* 中國中醫古籍總目. The text divides pharmaceutical drugs into 9 groups: 玉石部, jade and minerals; 草部上中下, herbs, upper,
middle, lower section; 木部, trees; 人部, man; 禽獸部, birds and quadrupeds;
蟲魚部, insects and fish; 果品部, fruits; 米穀部, rice and cereals; 蔬菜部, vegetables. A comparison shows that the contents of this volume were copied from
the Ming author Luo Biwei's 羅必煒 *Yi fang yao xing*'s 醫方藥性 first *juan*: Yao
xing fu zhi jie 藥性賦直解. However, in Luo's book, the rhymed verses are accompanied by explanatory notes on each substance. In the present volume,
these notes were omitted. Also, the present text is not entirely identical with
the source text. The original printing of the *Yi fang yao xing* – Yao xing fu zhi jie
醫方藥性·藥性賦直解 was produced rather carelessly and is marred by numer-
ous errors. As the copyist responsible for the present volume appears to have
had an outstanding level of education, and his calligraphy was first class, he
introduced corrections where he may have considered this necessary.

***

TITLE:            (*Fu zhou jue pu* 符咒訣譜, Instruction manual on charms
                  and spells)
ID:               8871
CONTENTS:         Exorcistic charms and oral spells
APPEARANCE:       Ancient manuscript volume. Cover and title page without
                  inscription. Good calligraphy.
BINDING:          Thread
MEASURE:          20 x 10.6
TITLE PAGE:       No
NO. OF PAGES:     32
L.P. /CH.L:       Numerous charms of different styles. Pages without such
                  drawings: 14 x approx. 28.

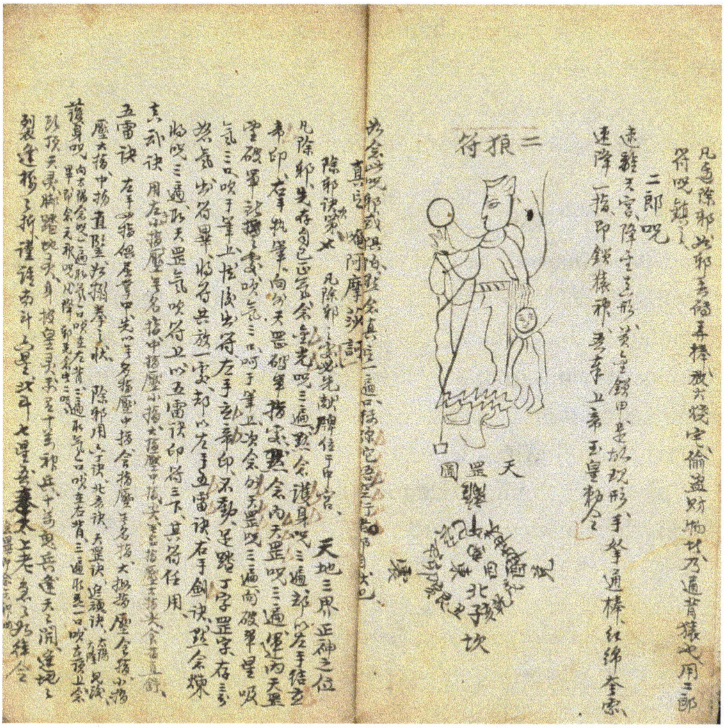

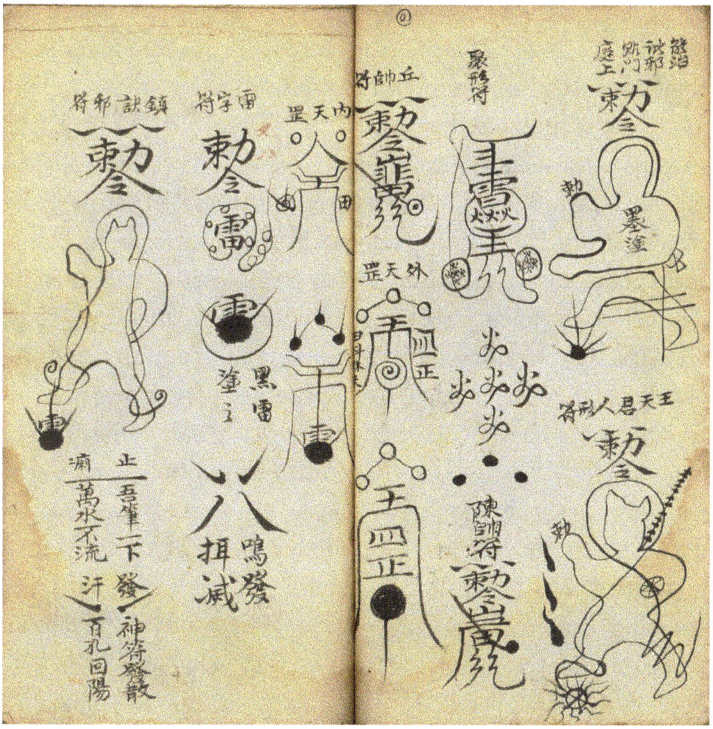

LAYOUT:              No lines, no frames
AUTHOR AND YEAR OF TEXT:
                     Unknown
YEAR OF COPY:    No observation of Qing dynasty taboos. Republican era.

SURVEY OF CONTENTS: This volume lists exorcistic charms and spells. It has
no preface. It begins with Bi xie fu 辟邪符, "Amulets to eliminate evil", Zhan
yao shu gui 斬妖殺鬼, "To behead goblins and to kill demons", Sha gui fu 煞
鬼符, "Amulets to kill demons". They are followed by San tian mi jue 三天秘
訣, "Secret instructions from the Three Heavens", a paragraph informing of the
pathological conditions to be discerned by identifying the demon responsible
for an illness. The following Xiang xie ge, 相邪歌, "Song to face evil", is a rhymed
discourse likewise helping to identify the type of demon responsible for an
ailment. Further sections include: 驅邪口訣及符式、遣鬼咒、二郎咒、天
罡圖、除邪訣、護身符、內天罡咒、遣邪咒、罩宅咒、門神咒、後門符、
東北鬼門符、王伯符、鎖邪符、運筆捉邪符、變化方形咒、招神將咒、遣
邪符（十餘種設計精巧的符式）、令牌（面式、背式）、雷印式、鎮病床
符、病人吞符、鐵牌符、帶符、臥床符、雷天咒、斬鬼神劍、除邪、（各
種劍的名稱及製法）、遣鬼破邪神劍咒、雷城十二門、馬元帥、溫元帥、
趙元帥、關元帥、尾火虎、井木犴、畢月烏、房日兔、翼火蛇、玄壇符、
遣邪合用（符式十餘道）. These are all apotropaic techniques to be resorted
to by magicians intending to exorcise demons.
　　A subsequent section has the title: 真獻大行法事化諸符治諸病. It includes
passages with titles such as Zhi xie fu zhou 治邪符咒, "Charm spells to cure
from evil", Zhi bing fu 治病符, "Charms to cure diseases". (They include dozens
of different charms. The majority are charm style charms; a smaller number
are Chinese characters style charms. These are all resorted to to treat illnesses.
Examples include diarrhea, *xie* 瀉; constipation of feces and urine, *da xiao bian
bu tong* 大小便不通; vomiting, *ou tu* 嘔吐; abdominal pain, *du teng* 肚疼, et al.);
Zhi zhong du zhu 治腫毒咒, "Spells to cure swelling poison"; Nei tian gang 內天
罡, "Star of the inner heaven"; Wai tian gang 外天罡, "Star of the outer heaven";
Chu xie qu sha fa 除邪取煞氣法, "Patterns to drive off evil and to catch demons"; Zhi bing qu sheng qi fa 治病取生氣法, "Patterns to cure diseases and to
acquire vital qi"; Zhi yin yang leng bing qu yang sheng fa 治陰陽冷病取養生法,
"Patterns to treat cold disease and to acquire and nourish vital [qi] by means
of yin and yang", Zhi re bing qu yang 33qi fa 治熱病取養氣法, "Patterns to treat
heat disease and to acquire and nourish [vital] qi"; Zhi fou fa 治痞法, "To cure
obstacle-illness"; Zhi xiao er ye ti、治小兒夜啼, "To cure weeping of children

during the night"; Cui sheng 催生, "To hasten delivery"; Nüe 瘧, "Malaria"; Yi qie za zheng 一切雜症, "Miscellaneous pathological conditions", E chuang 惡瘡, "Malign ulcers", etc.

Towards the end of the volume a section with the title Jue pu 訣譜, "Manual of instructions", lists about 30 to 40 different finger gestures used to achieve apotropaic ends. This is an unusually comprehensive listing.

In general, this volume might be identified as recording charms and spells as used by Daoist masters. However, the extent of documenting spells and finger gestures for the treatment of disease makes it rather special.

***

| | |
|---|---|
| TITLE: | (*Zhi fan zhen xie* 治犯鎮邪, To bring to order/cure opposition and suppress the evil) |
| ID: | 8872 |
| CONTENTS: | Charms and spells |
| APPEARANCE: | A rather unique ancient manuscript volume designed according to the vertical shape of charms. An account book is filled with charms in such a way that the spine of the book faces upward. For leafing through the volume, each page is to be turned upward. Hence the unusual measures of 21.3 cm height and 7.5 cm broadness. Brown kraft paper cover. No book title. |
| BINDING: | Thread |
| MEASURE: | 21.3 x 7.5 |
| TITLE PAGE: | No |
| NO. OF PAGES: | 46 |
| L.P. /CH.L: | No lines, no frames |
| LAYOUT: | Mostly one charm per page. |
| AUTHOR AND YEAR OF TEXT: | |
| | Unknown |
| YEAR OF COPY: | No Qing dynasty taboos observed. Republican era. |

SURVEY OF CONTENTS: The first page states: 治犯鎮邪, 解救良民. "To cure from the bad and suppress the evil, to rescue the good people." This is meant to express the function of charms and spells.

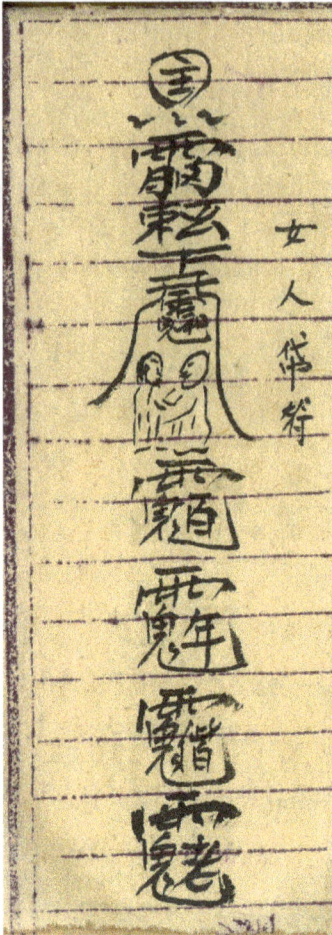

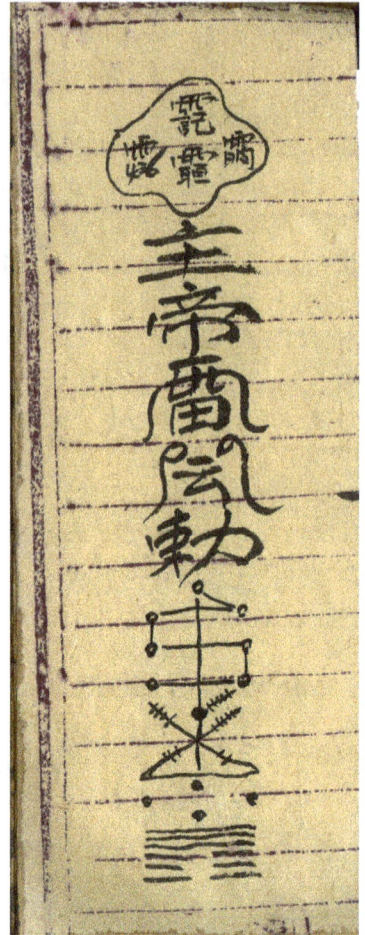

The volume has two parts, a Shang ji 上集, "upper collection", and a Xia ji 下集, "lower collection". However, it cannot be read like a normal illustrated volume. Rather, the "upper collection" is found by reading all front pages. To consult the "lower collection", the volume is to be turned around, and the back side of the pages are to be read.

The "upper collection" lists the following charms and spells: Zhen fan fe fu 鎮犯飛符; Zhen wu fang su sha fu 鎮五方三煞符; Bao fan fu 報犯符; Zhi shan xiao men shang tie 治山肖門上貼, a charm "to cure [illness caused by the demon] shan xiao, to be pasted on the door"; Zhi hu li jing zhang shang tie 治狐狸精帳上貼, a charm "to cure fox essence, to be pasted on the screen"; Qu xie fu 驅邪符; Fu zhen jiu zhou long hu fu 符鎮九洲龍虎伏; fa xing si hai gui shen jing 法行四海鬼神驚, a "charm to suppress dragons and tigers in the nine continents, and the method to horrify demons and spirits in the four seas." Zhi yao guai zhan fu 治妖怪戰符; Zhi bing fang men tie fu 治病房門貼符 (a charm shaped like a snake, "to be pasted on the door of the patient's room"); Huang quan fu 黃泉符; Zao xiang shui tui chao re shi 造香水退潮熱食; Lei shan fu wu dao 雷山符五道; Liu jia tai mu dai fu 六甲胎母帶符; Shuai zhang men jiang 帥帳門將; Fang men 房門; Liu jia ding fu 六甲釘符; San jie xie mo jie gong shou 三界邪魔皆拱手; Shi fang dao xi gui yi 十方外道悉皈依, "All to be converted in ten directions on the roads outside."

The contents of the "lower collection" are as follows: Liu jia an tai fu 六甲安胎符; Fan tai shen san dao 犯胎神三道; Xiao er ye ti hong zhi hua tie du qi 小兒夜啼紅紙花貼肚臍; Xiao er chu wai dai fu 小兒除外帶符; Zhi bai hu zhong sang fu 致白虎重喪符; Zhi sang che bai hu fu 致喪車白虎符; Zhi zhong fu san sang shu fu 致重伏三喪樹符; Cang shen fu 藏身符; Shan shui fu 山水符; Xi jiao nei tie fu 喜驕內貼符; Jiao men san shang 轎門傘上; Xin ren san shang 新人傘上; Song jia ren dai 送嫁人帶; Xin ren dai fu 新人帶符; Nü ren dai fu 女人帶符; Jia hui zi tu nei zhang gai xin ren 加諱字涂內藏蓋新人; Zhi dian shi fu 治癲食符; Ma Yuan shi meng zhong chuan fu shi 馬元帥夢中傳符食; Yang da xin fu 樣大新符; Fan huo xing fu 犯火星符.

***

TITLE:              (Fu zhou 符咒, Charms and spells)
ID:                 8873, 8874

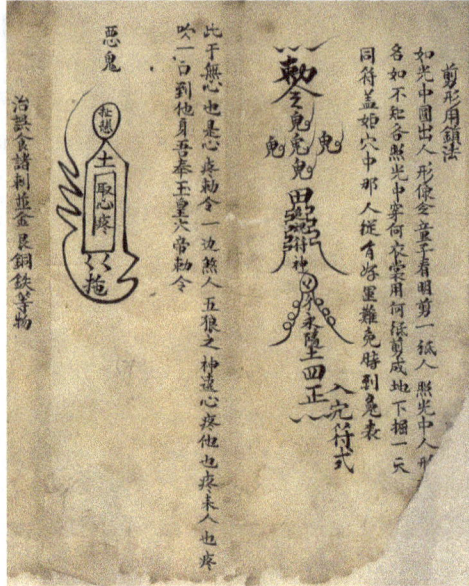

CONTENTS:        Charms and spells

APPEARANCE:      Two scrolls, without wooden axis, prepared from the pag-
                 es of a single book that was taken apart, with the separate
                 pages then glued to each other consecutively. Color slightly
                 yellowed. Careful handwriting. Calligraphy above average.

BINDING:         Not applicable

MEASURE:         Scroll 1: 26.0 x 253.5. Scroll 2: 26.0 x 371.0.

TITLE PAGE:      No. No title

NO. OF PAGES:    Not applicable

L.P. /CH.L:      26 characters/line

LAYOUT:          No lines, no frames

AUTHOR AND YEAR OF TEXT:

                 Anonymous. Qing dynasty

YEAR OF COPY:    Character 玄 occasionally written with final stroke omitted,
                 ocassionally written in complete form. The text has a Qing
                 dynasty *daoguang* 道光 reign period date (1820-1850). Pre-
                 sumably it was written at the end of the Qing dynasty to the
                 early Republican era.


SURVEY OF CONTENTS: These scrolls are Daoist records of charms and spells
of a widely diverse nature. Unlike most other texts on apotropaic approaches
they are not limited to exorcisms designed to cure illness.

The first scroll begins with sections Gai gui ya teng 蓋鬼牙疼, "To eliminate [lit: cover] demon toothache", and Zhi nü ren xin kou teng 治女人心口疼, "To cure pain in the heart/stomach opening of women" – with the characters for "heart opening", *xin kou* 心口, possibly used for "stomach opening", i.e., cardia, here. All the following charms are designed as calls to spirits. Three of the charms are rarely seen drawings of human figures, holding a weapon in their hands. The scroll ends with a request by a believer, dated in the *dao guang* 道光 reign period, directed at Yu huang da di 玉皇大帝, The Great Thearch of the Jade Augustus, to help to arrest a robber.

The second scroll contains numerous charms with symbolic design and used, for example, to call back a *hun* soul, to make someone feel dizzy, to summon a robber, to subdue a fire. Charms used to cure illness are mostly designed by using ordinary Chinese characters.

The second scroll's most conspicuous content is the "art of nightmare subjugation", *yan fu shu* 魘伏術. The demons visualized in a nightmare are transformed into images made of wood or dough, which then themselves are used as charms. This technique has been transmitted as a folk tradition. An example is the following "method to cut a physical appearance", *jian xing fa* 剪形法: 用桃木條三寸長，身穿青衣，插頭安足，做成人形。將某人年庚姓名硃字一條粘 于胸前，穿衣遮之，入于行法家震地溝渠之間，入地一尺，紙人腰間包符入之。"Take a three-inches long peach wood twig. The body wears a virid clothing. Stick in a head and put feet in their place to form a human figure. Use vermilion to write a person's birthdates and name on a paper slip to be glued to the chest [of that figure]. Cover it with the clothing. The person applying this technique is then to bury it near a ditch by the house at a *Zhen*-hexagram/earth spot; 1 *chi* deep into the earth. The charm is to be wrapped around the waist of the paper effigy." This is accompanied by a charm drawing.

An example for using dough rather than wood is the "method to form a figure by kneading dough", *nie mian zuo xing fa* 捏麵作形法, documented in the 2nd scroll: 用麵人一個作成，將血馀灰插滿頭中，赤身不衣，背面具書某人姓名元形，心口窩寫一心字，用針刺之。耳目口鼻但要針開一下，用符一道，包著麵人，咒曰：吾奉太乙真沉元喪爾魂，晏公揮爾首，取王焚爾身，五龍并小聖波回淪元塵去，敕。用劍訣。"Prepare a human figurine from dough. Cover the entire head with ashes obtained from burning hair. The body remains naked without clothing. Write that person's name and describe his/her physical appearance on the figurine's back. Write a single character *xin* ["heart"] on the figurine's stomach pit and pierce it with a needle. Ears, eyes, mouth and nose must be opened by means of a needle. Take a charm [written on paper] and wrap it around the dough figurine. The spell says: "I beg Tai yi zhen Chen Yuan to kill your *hun*-spirit, Yan gong to wipe off your head, Qu Wang to burn your body, Wu long and Xiao sheng po hui lun .. (final characters remain unclear). Imperial command. To be applied with sword gestures".

Attached is a *bao mian ren fu shi* 包麵人符式, "Amulet model for wrapping around a human figurine made of dough". An explanatory note says: 此符包著麵人，往坎水河中送下去，來不回頭, "This human figurine made of dough with the charm wrapped around is to be discarded by going to the river as a *Kan*-hexamgram/water spot. One goes away and must not turn his head." Another *qu xin teng fa* 取心疼法, "Method to make use of pain in the heart" is also an example of an application of the *yan fu fa* 魘伏法, method to "subjugate nightmares". By piercing the charm with a needle, an enemy is supposed to be made suffering of pain in his heart.

Examples of the many written character-type charms designed to cure illnesses are *zhi wu shi zhu ci bing jin yin tong tie deng wu* 治誤食諸刺并金銀銅鐵等物, "To cure [illness resulting from] an erroneous consumption of thorns and all items made of gold, silver, copper and iron"; *jin gu teng tong gao yao* 筋骨疼痛膏藥, "Oint medication for sinew and bone pain", and *xie zhe shen fang* 蝎蜇神方, "Divine recipe for scorpion stings".

The 2ⁿᵈ scroll has two requests directed at the "Lord of the Kitchen Range", *zao jun* 皂（灶）君, to search for a robber. Here the region Lai zhou 萊州 in Shandong 山東 province and a date in the *dao guang* 道光 reign period (1820-1850) are mentioned. From these entries it is possible to identify the origin of this scroll and the time of its preparation.

\*\*\*

| | |
|---|---|
| TITLE: | *Yin pian jia mu zong lu* 飲片價目總錄, Complete price list of herbal tablets |
| ID: | 8875 |
| CONTENTS: | Materia medica |
| APPEARANCE: | Small, pocket-size leporello-format manuscript volume. Calligraphy above average. Front page with inscription |
| BINDING: | Not applicable |
| MEASURE: | 12.2 x 5.0 |
| TITLE PAGE: | Yes. Inscription on the left: 飲片價目總錄/首. In the center: 民國元年十二月二十日吉立. |

NO. OF PAGES:        52
L.P. /CH.L:          3 horizontal columns. 5 characters per column.
LAYOUT:              No lines, no frames
AUTHOR AND YEAR OF TEXT:
                     Some pharmacist, 1st year Republican era: 1912.
YEAR OF COPY:        The inscription on the title page identifies this volume as
                     written in 1912. As this was just the beginning of the Repub-
                     lican era, the written text continues many times the taboos
                     imposed on certain characters during the Qing dynasty.

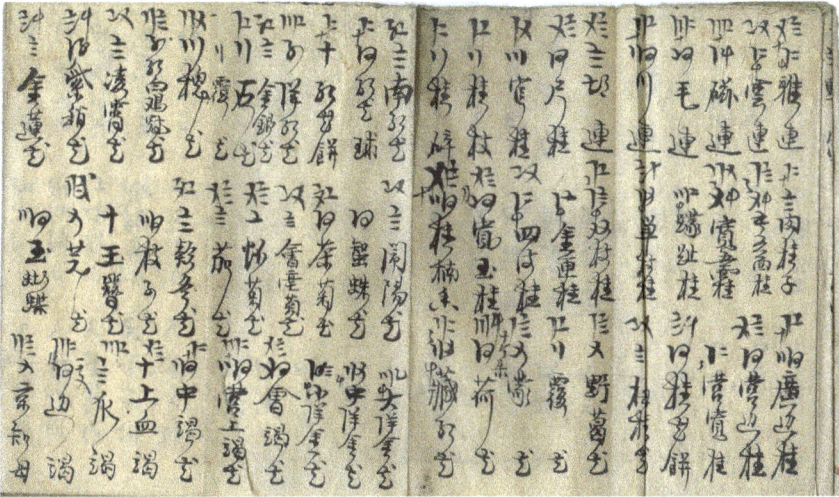

SURVEY OF CONTENTS: This is a price list of 750 items of traditional herbal
medicine prepared for use as a decoction (*zhong yao yin pian* 中藥飲片), dated 1912. Above each medication's name the price is given, written with "orna-
mental numbers", *hua ma* 花碼. The names are those popular at the time and
they are not standardized yet. Thus, one identical herbal drug may be listed
under different names. An example is *da huang* 大黃. In the present volume
it is mentioned with 9 different names: *ye jun* 野軍, *xi ning jun* 西寧軍, *jin wen
jun* 錦紋軍, *min zhong ji* 岷中吉, *da huang ban* 大黃办（瓣）, *da huang mian*
大黃面, *chuan tai da huang* 川台大黃, *jiu jun* 酒軍, and *jiu jun* 炙軍. Hence this
volume is not only a valuable source for researching the prices of traditional
herbal medicines during the Republican era. It also offers rich data on the designations of these medicines at the end of the Qing dynasty and in the early
Republican era.

***

TITLE: *Zhi ma bing fang dai ge. Yao wu ju* 治馬病方帶歌·藥物劇,
Song on recipes for curing horses, to be carried at the girdle.
Drama with pharmaceutical drugs

ID: 8876

CONTENTS:        Veterinary medicine. Entertainment
APPEARANCE:      Large format ancient manuscript volume. Margins and edg-
                 es considerably damaged. Average calligraphy in a first part
                 devoted to veterinary medicine. Excellent calligraphy in the
                 second part devoted to a folk opera libretto.
BINDING:         Thread
MEASURE:         21.2 x 23.0
TITLE PAGE:      Lost. First page with table of contents of veterinary medi-
                 cine part.
NO. OF PAGES:    Vet. med. section: 25, Opera libretto: 15
L.P. /CH.L:      Vet. med. section: 16 x 25, Opera libretto: 16 x 35
LAYOUT:          No lines, no frames
AUTHOR AND YEAR OF TEXT:
                 Unknown, Qing dynasty
YEAR OF COPY:    Characters 玄 and 寧 written to observe Qing dynasty ta-
                 boos. Qing dynasty.

SURVEY OF CONTENTS: This volume consists of two parts, written by different
hands. The first part is Zhi ma bing fang dai ge 治馬病方帶歌. We give a tentative title Yao wu ju 藥物劇, "Pharmaceutical drama", to the second part.

The first part has 72 recipe entries divided along illnesses affecting the five
long-term depots, and miscellaneous treatments. Under each recipe's name
are listed the therapeutic indication, the composition (without quantities of
individual constituents), the method of ingestion, and a rhymed recipe. These
recipes are followed by another list of 13 recipes with identical structure of
the text but without the rhymed part. In contrast to other such manuals, the
present volume does not offer drawings of diseased horses. The recipes listed
are all those with many ingredients. The text does not mention a single recipe
with only one constituent.

The opera libretto is recorded here without title. We have given it a tentative
title in view of the contents of other such volumes. The present drama has 10
scenes. They differ from the scenes in other such librettos.

1st scene:   甘國老請醫敘寒, Gan Guolao asks a physician to explain to him
             "cold"
2nd scene:   佳人誣犯彌陀僧, a beautiful woman falsely accuses the priest Mi
             tuo
3rd scene:   山梔子投熱遇妖, Shan Zhizi turns hot and encounters a goblin
4th scene:   路旁幸遇馬齒莧, at the road-side luckily meets Ma Chixian

5<sup>th</sup> scene: 威靈仙溫村顯武, Wei Lingxian in the village Wen shows his military skills

6<sup>th</sup> scene: 紅娘子賣藥被戲耍, Miss Hong is made fun of when purchasing medicine

7<sup>th</sup> scene: 石決明得病招禍端, Shi Jueming falls ill and calls on the origin of his calamity

8<sup>th</sup> scene: 海桐決明大交鋒, Hai Tong and Jue Ming engage in a massive battle

9<sup>th</sup> scene: 南天星奉旨使平亂, Nan Tianxing receives an imperial decree to calm down the disturbance

10<sup>th</sup> scene: 茯苓神營前主婚配, God Fu Ling presides over the wedding ceremony in front of the camp.

Thus, the drama recorded in this volume is entirely different from those found in other volumes.

The volume concludes with several poems that are not related to medicine.

***

TITLE: *Zhu you ke zhu fu mi jue. Tian yi shi san ke zhi bing yi zong* 祝由科諸符秘訣·天醫十三科治病一宗, Secret instructions on all types of charms from the [therapeutic] specialty of invocation of the origin. The lineage of celestial physicians of the thirteenth specialty that cure disease.

ID: 8877

CONTENTS: Exorcism

APPEARANCE: Ancient manuscript volume without title. Excellent calligraphy.

BINDING: Paper spills

MEASURE: 24.0 x 14.6

TITLE PAGE: No. No table of contents

NO. OF PAGES: 50

L.P. /CH.L: Approx. 8 x 15

LAYOUT: No lines, no frames

AUTHOR AND YEAR OF TEXT:

Anonymous, Qing dynasty

YEAR OF COPY: Paper quality suggests Republican era.

SURVEY OF CONTENTS: This is a regular exorcist manual for therapeutic purposes. It has two parts: Zhu you ke zhu fu mi jue 祝由科諸符秘訣, and Tian yi shi san ke zhi bing yi zong 天醫十三科治病一宗.

The first section relies for the most part on written character-style charms. For each such charm the illness it may cure is named. Most of these character-style charms have the character *shang* 尚 as their header. The therapeutic indications include 疔瘡腫毒、傷寒、女人經脈不調、心痛痞塊、虎傷、蛇傷、狗咬、破傷風、痔漏、瘧疾、心痛、難產、惡瘡等. They are followed by mostly graphic charms, interspersed by written-character-style charms. They are not so much recommended for treating illnesses but for eliminating mosquitoes and curing injuries caused by animals. The text also lists very many oral spells.

The section Tian yi shi san ke zhi bing yi zong 天醫十三科治病一宗 focusses on charms designed to stimulate specific physician-immortals/"celestial physicians" of 13 specialties to cure an illness. Hence it may be identified as an example of regular medical-exorcism texts. The text begins with a Qing tian yi xin xiang fu 請天醫信香符. An explanatory note states: "This charm serves to let true incense descend. Write the charm in the middle. On both sides write the oral spell. Burn the incense in an oven. Kneel down to voice the prayer," *ci fu yong jiang zhen xiang, zhong jian shu fu, liang bian xie zhou yu, fan xiang lu nei,*

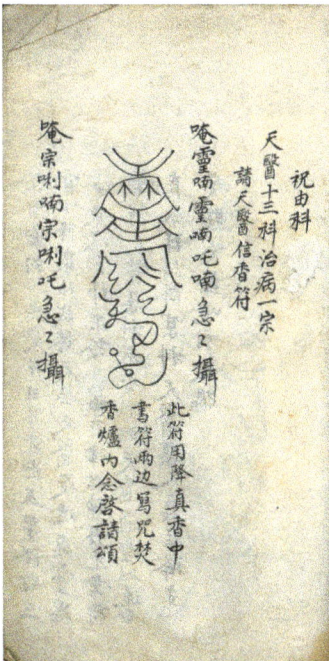

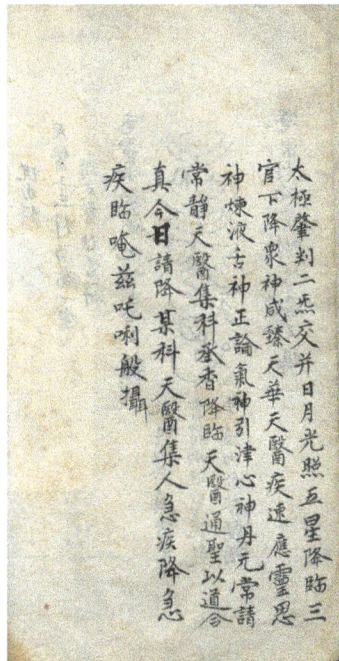

*nian qi qing song* 此符用降真香，中間書符，兩邊寫咒語，焚香爐內，念啓
請頌.

The subsequent sequence of charms is as follows:

召風科天醫符: charm to call on the Celestial Physicians of Wind Specialty
召大方脈天醫符: charm to call on the Celestial Physicians of Adult Medicine
召眼科天醫符: charm to call on the Celestial Physicians of Ophthalmology
召產科天醫符: charm to call on the Celestial Physicians of Obstetrics.
召外科天醫符: charm to call on the Celestial Physicians of the External Specialty
召小兒科天醫符: charm to call on the Celestial Physicians of Pediatrics
召耳鼻科天醫符: charm to call on the Celestial Physicians of the Ear/Nose Specialty
召齒牙科天醫符: charm to call on the Celestial Physicians of the Dental Specialty
召傷折科天醫符: charm to call on the Celestial Physicians of Traumatology
召金簇科天醫符: charm to call on the Celestial Physicians of the Specialty concerned with [wounds inflicted by] Metal Arrowheads
召砭針科天醫符: charm to call on the Celestial Physicians of Acupuncture Specialty
召瘡腫科天醫符: charm to call on the Celestial Physicians of Ulcer and Swelling Specialty
召書禁科天醫符: charm to call on the Celestial Physicians of the Specialty of Writing Spells.

In each instance, the names of the relevant "celestial physicians" are specified.

This is followed by a list of 14 charms designed to treat illnesses of various types. For example, referred to as "Medical Specialty for Diseases affecting Adults", *da fang mai ke* 大方脈科, a charm to cure heart and spleen pain is recommended. In most cases they are to be ingested with a pharmaceutical decoction.

***

TITLE:         *Zu chuan mi fang quan shu* 祖傳秘方全書, Complete book of secret recipes transmitted by the ancestors
ID:            8878
CONTENTS:      Pharmaceutical recipes

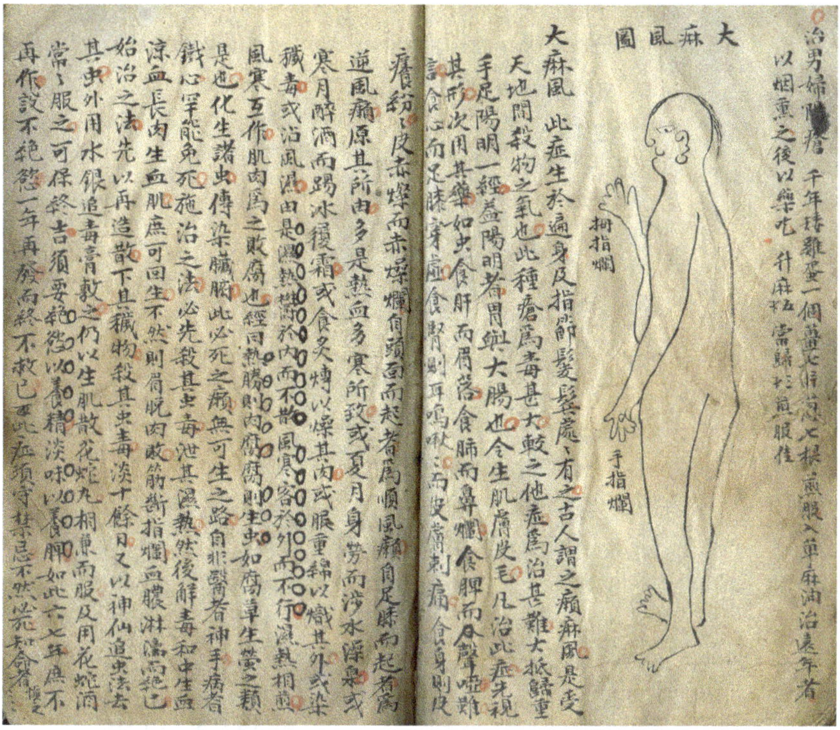
大痲風圖
拇指爛
手指爛

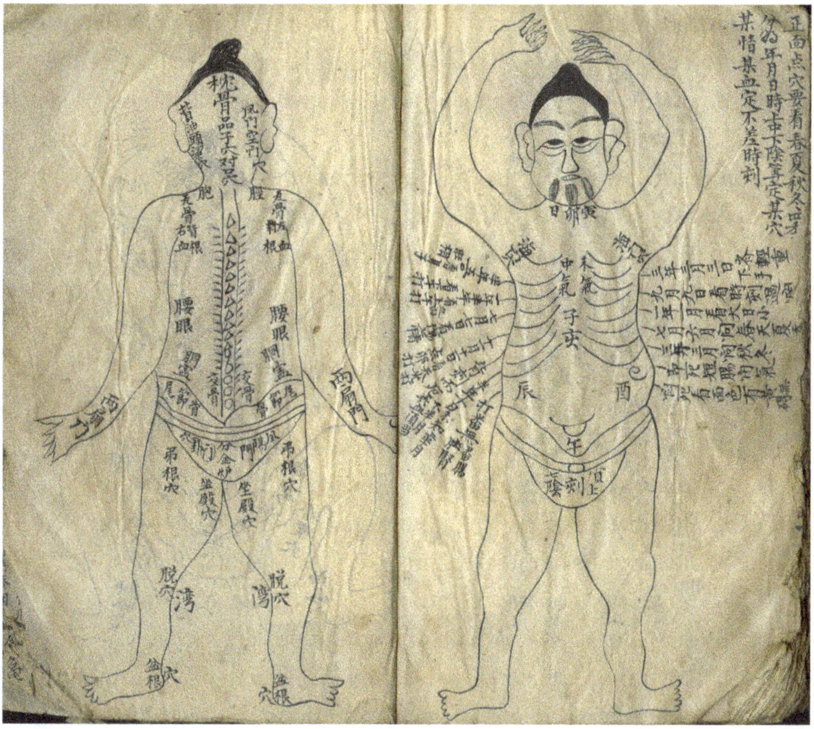
腰眼
吊根穴
生殿穴
辰
酉
午

APPEARANCE: Severely damaged ancient manuscript volume. Thick cover prepared from various layers of paper glued to each other; surface coarse and wrinkled. Three vertical inscriptions from left to right: 祖傳秘方全書/李時方立/乾隆四年. They may have been added by later hand, and cannot necessarily be trusted. Average calligraphy.

BINDING: Thread

MEASURE: 21.8 x 14.1

TITLE PAGE: No

NO. OF PAGES: 107

L.P. /CH.L: 10 x 30

LAYOUT: No lines, no frames

AUTHOR AND YEAR OF TEXT:

Anoymous, Qing dynasty

YEAR OF COPY: Character 玄 not written to observe a Qing dynasty taboo. Republican era.

SURVEY OF CONTENTS: This is a record of about 200 pharmaceutical recipes. Its contents may have been copied from printed books. They are partly identical with those of another manuscript volume, 8904, with the title *Wai ke ju zheng yao fang quan tu* 外科舉症藥方全圖. A special feature of the present volume are drawings of human bodies showing the locations of specific pathological conditions. The subsequent text then explains these conditions and recommendes pharmaceutical substances for their treatment.

The sequence of sections is as follows:

Tiao zhi yong du yao fang 調治癰毒藥方, "Pharmaceutical recipes to regulate and cure obstruction-illness poison", listing 36 recipes.

七症圖, "illustrations of seven pathological conditions", listing 50 recipes.

九症圖, "illustrations of nine pathological conditions",

十二症圖, "illustrations of twelve pathological conditions", 31 recipes.

十四症圖, "illustrations of fourteen pathological conditions", 33 recipes.

十二症圖, "illustrations of twelve pathological conditions", 16 recipes.

十二症圖, "illustrations of twelve pathological conditions", 14 recipes.

十五症圖, "illustrations of fifteen pathological conditions", 28 recipes.

十一症圖, "illustrations of eleven pathological conditions", 5 recipes.

五症圖, "illustrations of five pathological conditions", 12 recipes.

大麻風圖, "illustrations of 'major numbing wind' [leprosy]", 6 recipes.

十症圖, "illustrations of ten pathological conditions", no recipes.

七症圖, "illustrations of seven pathological conditions",
Many of these recipes are listed in other manuscript volumes, too.

This section is followed by a section An tai cui sheng yao fang 安胎催生藥方, "recipes to calm down the fetus and hasten delivery", transmitted by a Mr. Li Cunren 李存仁. It lists more than 100 recipes from the arena of gynecology.

*\*\**

| TITLE: | (*Ling yi lun bing chu fang* 鈴醫論病處方, A rattle healer's discourse on illnesses and recipes) |
|---|---|
| ID: | 8879 |
| CONTENTS: | Itinerant healer's records |
| APPEARANCE: | Large size ancient manuscript volume. Original cover and first part missing. New cover added by later hand: brocade pasted on paper. No title. Average calligraphy. |
| BINDING: | Thread |
| MEASURE: | 27.1 x 19.6 |
| TITLE PAGE: | No |
| NO. OF PAGES: | 33 |
| L.P. /CH.L: | 10 x 19 |
| LAYOUT: | No lines, no frames |

AUTHOR AND YEAR OF TEXT:
　　　　　　　Anonymous, End of Qing dynasty
YEAR OF COPY:　No Qing dynasty taboos observed. Presumably Republican
　　　　　　　era copy of mostly Qing dynasty contents.

SURVEY OF CONTENTS: This manuscript volume has the richest contents of all such volumes concerning a discussion of illnesses. Because in its present condition it has no cover and title page, and since the beginning pages are missing, the original title and the author remain unknown. The first half of this volume focusses on a discussion of illnesses. The second half is a list of pharmaceutical recipes.

The illnesses treated in the first half include: 咳嗽 *ke sou*, "cough"; 肚內寒症 *du nei han zheng*, "illness signs of abdominal cold"; 眼疼 *yan teng*, "aching eyes"; 婦人經血之症 *fu ren jing xue zheng*, "illness signs of women associated with menstrual bleeding"; 肩膀疼 *jian bang teng*, "aching shoulders"; 臌悶脹痛 *gu men zhang tong*, "drum-like distension, heart-pressure, swelling and pain"; 疔毒惡瘡 *ding du e chuang*, "Pin-illness poison with malign sores"; 夜夢遺精 *ye meng yi jing*, "night dream with involuntary loss of sperma". Further discourses are: 醫生論 Yi sheng lun, "On physicians"; 三關九殼（竅） San guan jiu qiao, "The three passes/joints and nine openings"; 五運六氣 wu yun liu qi, "The five periods and six qi"; 用藥之理 Yong yao zhi li, "Principles of drug use"; 診脈 Zhen mai, "Examination of the [movements in the] vessels"; 行針法 Xing zhen fa, "Methods of needling"; 高緩歷史 Gao huan li shi, "History of [the physician] Gao Huan; 一般醫理 Yi ban yi li, "General principles of medicine"; 七言歌訣 Qi yan ge jue, "Rhymed instructions in seven words".

Apparently, almost one half of the text on illnesses is missing. Following the section 夜夢遺精 a note says "The 18 major conditions [treated] above." *yi shang shi ba zheng* 以上十八大症. However, in the present volume only eight conditions are discussed; the pages on the remaining ten conditions are lost.

At first glance the discourse appears to be based in regular Chinese medical theory. The fact is, in many respects the conditions are exaggerated, misrepresented, and mixed with folk knowledge and legends. Such medical theory as proposed by itinerant physicians constitutes the most valuable part of this volume. The erroneous writing of the character *qiao* 竅 as 壳 shows that this is a volume written by an itinerant physician in the North of China.

The second half lists 58 pharmaceutical recipes. They include neither faked drugs nor those considered by itinerant physicians to act as *ding* 頂, *chuan* 串, *jie* 截, and *jin* 禁. On the contrary, they are not different from those used in regular Chinese medicine. Not surprisingly, they include recipes for abortion, such as a *cui tai san* 催胎散, "powder to hasten a fetus", and *duan tai san* 斷胎散, "powder to cut off a fetus". A "recipe to make one abstain from opium", *ji da yan fang* 計（忌）大煙方, must have originated in the late Qing dynasty period.

The text concludes with a section "To pierce evil. Secret essentials", Zhen xie mi yao 針邪秘要. This is an example of an amalgamation of exorcism and acupuncture. The illnesses suggested for such treatments appear to be mostly those identified as psychiatric diseases nowadays.

***

| | |
|---|---|
| TITLE: | *Fu Qingzhu nü ke* 傅青主女科, Fu Qingzhu's gynecology |
| ID: | 8880 |
| CONTENTS: | Gynecology |
| APPEARANCE: | Ancient manuscript volume of rare quality. Careful handwriting. Excellent calligraphy. Cover: tough paper made from bast fibre of the paper mulberry. Upper left, inscription: 傅青主女科. Lower right, inscription: 邢尚志. The character 傅 is erroneously written 傳. Also, the style of writing differs from the main text. Hence the inscriptions appear to have been added by later hand. |
| BINDING: | Thread |
| MEASURE: | 19.7 x 11.6 |
| TITLE PAGE: | No |
| NO. OF PAGES: | 65 |
| L.P. /CH.L: | 8 x 20 |
| LAYOUT: | No lines, no frames. Occasionally notes and commentaries written in small characters at the top of a page. |
| AUTHOR AND YEAR OF TEXT: | |
| | Fu Qingzhu 傅青主, ca. 1684. |
| YEAR OF COPY: | No Qing dynasty taboos observed. Republican era. |

SURVEY OF CONTENTS: The text begins with three paragraphs. The first is Yuan xu 原序, "Original preface". It is signed 道光丁亥夏五月丹崖張鳳翔題. The second is Nü ke kao lüe 女科考略, "An outline of gynecology". It is signed 道光十一年新正上元同里後學祈爾誠謹序. The third has the heading Xu 序, "Preface". It is signed: 咸豐元年正月上元日太原孟先穎又章氏謹識. In his preface Mr. Meng states: 自張丹崖廣文初刻於太原，祁竹崖刺史再刻於都門. This shows that the present volume was copied from an 1851 printed edition.

The volume is designed like a printed book. At the beginning a table of contents states: 共三十八條，三十九症，四十一方, "[This book] comprises 38 paragraphs with 39 illness signs and 41 recipes". The heading at the beginning

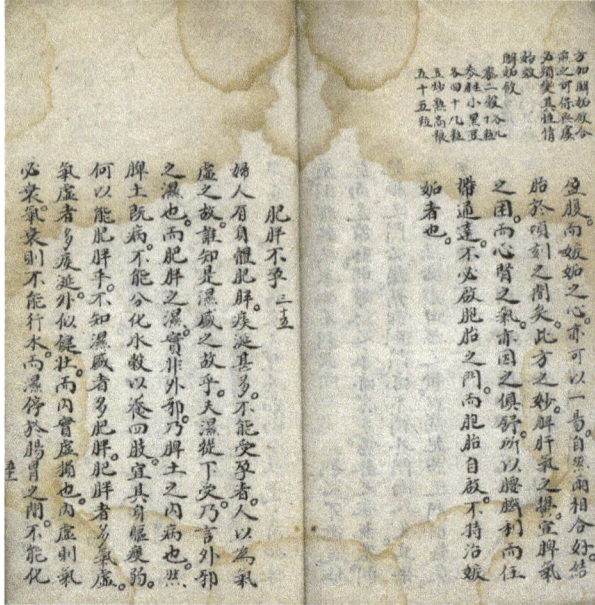

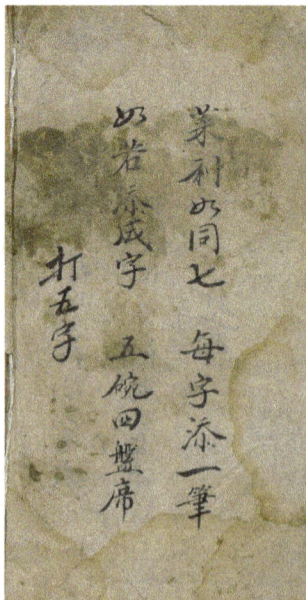

of the main text was changed from 女科卷一, "gynecology, first *juan*", to 女科卷 全, "gynecology, complete *juan*". To the very end of the main text were added the two characters 卷終, "end of *juan*". According to the table of contents, there should have existed a second volume. It is not present in this collection.

\*\*\*

TITLE: *Fan ke* 範科, *Fan* (?) specialty
ID: 8881
CONTENTS: Pediatrics
APPEARANCE: Ancient manuscript volume of poor quality. Calligraphy above average. Cover made of tough paper prepared from the bast fibre of the paper mulberry, added by later hand in addition to the remaining original cover. Upper left, inscription: 範科, with upper half of character 範 destroyed. Lower left, inscription: 羅國泉氏. This is the name of the copyist.
BINDING: Thread
MEASURE: 19.2 x 11.5
TITLE PAGE: No
NO. OF PAGES: 19
L.P. /CH.L: 8 x approx. 23
LAYOUT: No lines, no frames
AUTHOR AND YEAR OF TEXT:
　　　　　　Author unknown. Copyist: Luo Guoquan 羅國泉
YEAR OF COPY: Character 玄 not written to observe a Qing dynasty taboo. Republican era.

SURVEY OF CONTENTS: This book focusses on folk lamp wick cauterization. Its first 22 half pages each show a human figure drawn in the upper half and an explanatory text written in the lower half. Red dots indicate the locations on a human person where such cauterization is to be applied for treating the specified conditions. The therapeutic indications treated here are all from the realm of pediatric fright conditions: 撮口急驚風、慢驚風、膨脹驚、鯽魚驚、夜啼驚、臍風驚、挽弓驚、胎驚、烏鴉驚、烏紗驚、月家驚、天吊驚、肚痛驚、看地驚、潮熱驚、蛇系驚、馬啼（蹄）驚、鷹爪驚、水泄驚、撒手驚、內吊驚、迷魂驚.

The latter part of this volume is a section Da xiao er jing zheng er shi si ge ju 大小兒驚症二十四歌訣, "Twenty four rhymed instructions on fright conditions of older and younger children," discussing the fright conditions listed earlier. However, the therapeutic approach advised here is *tui na* 推拿 push-and-pull massage rather than lampwick cauterization.

The volume concludes with a section Zeng bu zhen mai zong mai 增補診脈 總脈, which offers simple instructions on pulse diagnosis.

YEAR OF COPY: Character 玄 not written to observe a Qing dynasty taboo. Republican era.

\*\*\*

TITLE: *Xian tian ba gua tu* 先天八卦圖, Illustrated eight trigrams and the [endowment by] heaven from previous [to one's existence]

ID: 8882

CONTENTS: Fortune telling

APPEARANCE: Dirty ancient manuscript volume. Cover darkened. Upper left, inscription: 先天八卦圖. Lower right, seal: 夏用寶印. Careful handwriting. Average calligraphy.

BINDING: Thread

MEASURE: 18.2 x 12.2

TITLE PAGE: Yes. Inscription: 先天八卦圖. Lower right, seal: 夏用寶印. Back of title page: heading 鬼老天. Below depiction of the names of the 8 trigrams and a Ying shan tu 塋山圖, "Grave hill" illustration.

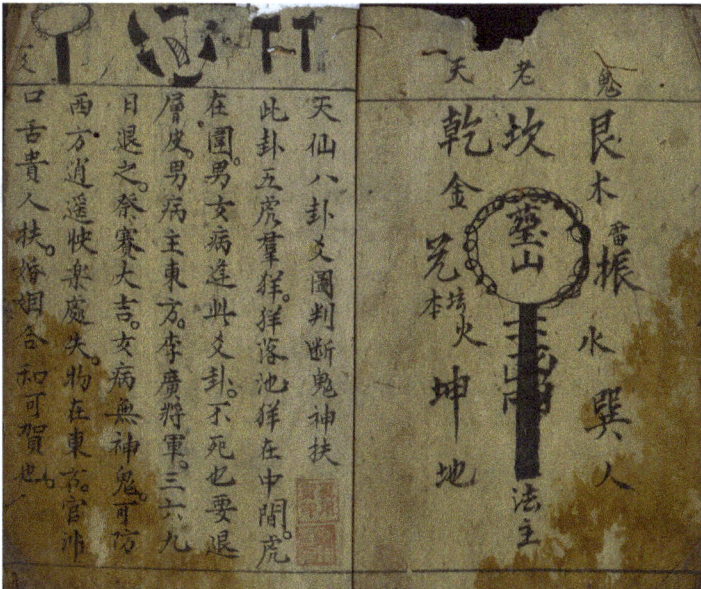

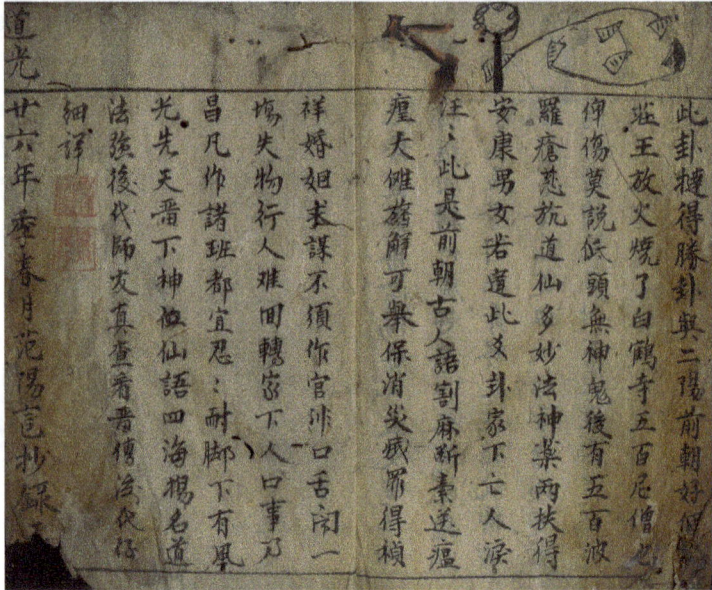

NO. OF PAGES:        24

L.P. /CH.L:          7 x 14

LAYOUT:              Upper and lower margins separated by line.

AUTHOR AND YEAR OF TEXT:

Author: anonymous. Copyist: Xia Yongbao 夏用寶. Qing dynasty.

YEAR OF COPY:  Inscription on final page: 道光廿六年季春范陽[言/己]抄錄. The character 玄 is written to observe a Qing dynasty taboo. Volume prepared in 1846.

SURVEY OF CONTENTS: This is a manual on an ancient technique of fortune telling. In the upper margins of each page a set of symbols (six black and white lines; two hatchets, one semi-circle) are drawn in varying arrangements. These arrangements are then identified as auspicious or inauspicious signs with regard to a person's travel plans, health, etc. The meaning of the symbols lines, hatchets and semi-circle, and the technique of generating the various arrangements remain unclear without consulting special literature.

***

TITLE: *Dao yuan jin jing* 道緣金鏡, Golden mirror of the *Dao*'s course.

ID: 8883

CONTENTS: Daoism

APPEARANCE: Ancient manuscript volume. Careful handwriting. Average calligraphy. Cover made from paper mulberry. Blank.

BINDING: Thread

MEASURE: 17.1 x 12.4

TITLE PAGE: Blank

NO. OF PAGES: 27

L.P. /CH.L: 9 x 16

LAYOUT: No lines, no frames

AUTHOR AND YEAR OF TEXT:

Anonymous, Qing dynasty.

YEAR OF COPY: No Qing dynasty taboos observed. Republican era.

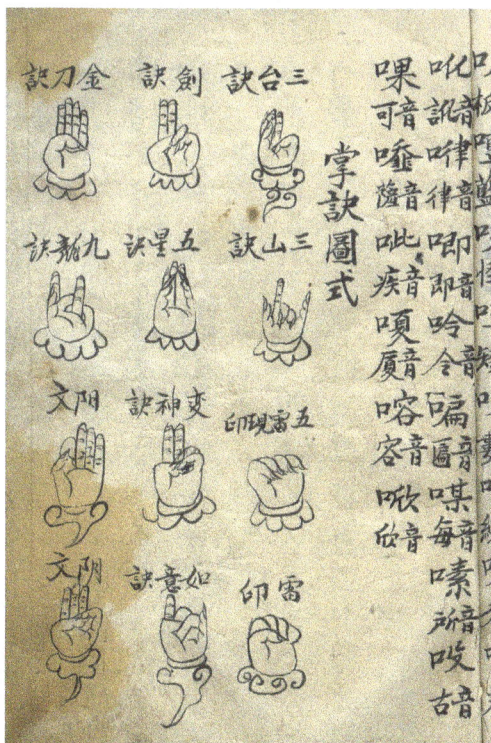

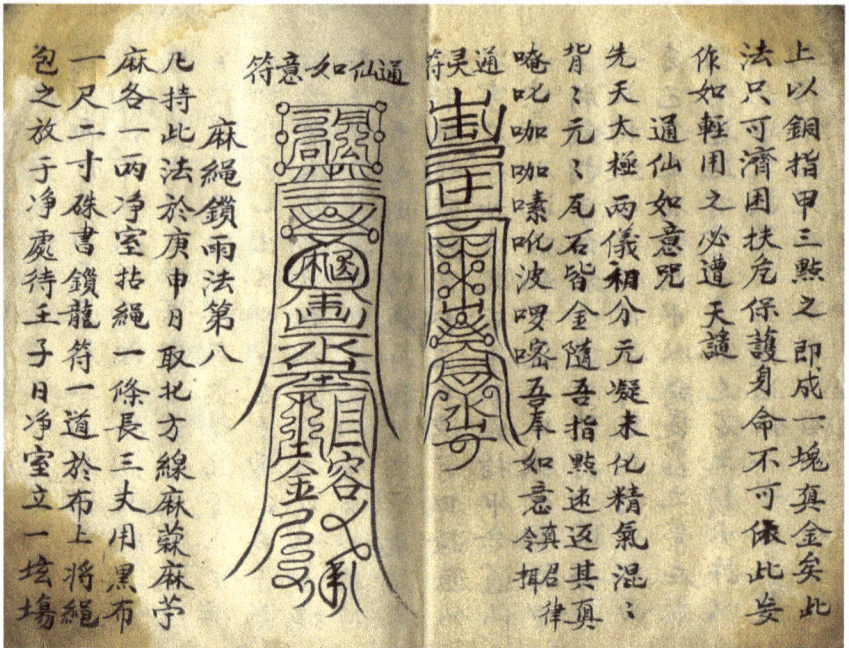

SURVEY OF CONTENTS: This is a text on Daoist techniques. It has a table of contents listing 18 paragraphs. The first is 洪濛隱家法第一. The final paragraph is 合和地仙丹第十八. Among the issues treated are: Bian hua shen xing fa 變化身形法, (This paragraph is mentioned in the table of contents but is absent from the main text), "A method to transform the human body"; Sa dou cheng bing fa 撒豆成兵法, "A method to drop beans to generate weapons"; An lu lian bao fa 安爐煉寶法, "To install an oven to refine a treasure", and Dian shi cheng jin fa 點石成金法, "A method to touch a stone and turn it into gold".

A section Qu chu han re fa 驅除寒熱法, "A method to drive away cold and heat", is related to health care, as are sections 10 through 18 introducing *dan* 丹, "elixir", medication, the so-called *Huang di jiu dan* 黃帝九丹, "Huang Di's nine elixirs". They include: 一氣混元丹、無極太元丹、三才固真丹、黃庭種子丹、子午交互丹、草還生生丹、返老還童丹、太乙乾元丹、合和地仙丹. Each of these "elixirs" requires a charm, an oral spell, and up to ten pharmaceutical substances. The application includes burning of the charms and ingestion of the pharmaceutical drugs. Such an approach is rarely documented.

In the final section of the volume a list of 150 characters, each written with the character *kou* 口 to its left, is offered together with their pronunciation. This section has the title Fo mu yin zi 佛母音字. The following section offers Zhang jue tu shi 掌訣圖式, "Drawings of manual instructions". These are 19 finger gestures to be shown by a practitioner performing his rituals.

\*\*\*

| TITLE: | *Yan fang wen jian lu. Za zheng.* 驗方聞見錄·雜証, Record of proven recipes heard of and seen. For miscellaneous signs [of disease] |
|---|---|
| ID: | 8884 |
| CONTENTS: | Pharmaceutical recipes |
| APPEARANCE: | Simple ancient manuscript volume, written by several different hands. Hence the handwriting differs and is fine in some parts and inferior in others. Cover made from paper mulberry paper. Red paper label with title written in black: 驗方聞見錄. Center, inscription directly on cover 雜証. Latter section of main text with punctuation marks. |
| BINDING: | Paper spills |
| MEASURE: | 19.2 x 13.8 |
| TITLE PAGE: | No |
| NO. OF PAGES: | 38 |
| L.P. /CH.L: | 8 x 20 |
| LAYOUT: | No lines, no frames |
| AUTHOR AND YEAR OF TEXT: | Unknown |
| YEAR OF COPY: | Some remarks on Western medicine are interspersed. Republican era. |

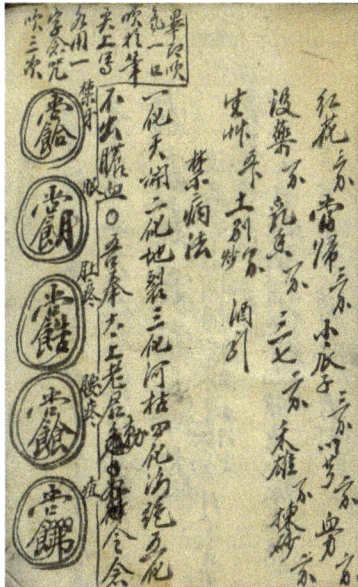

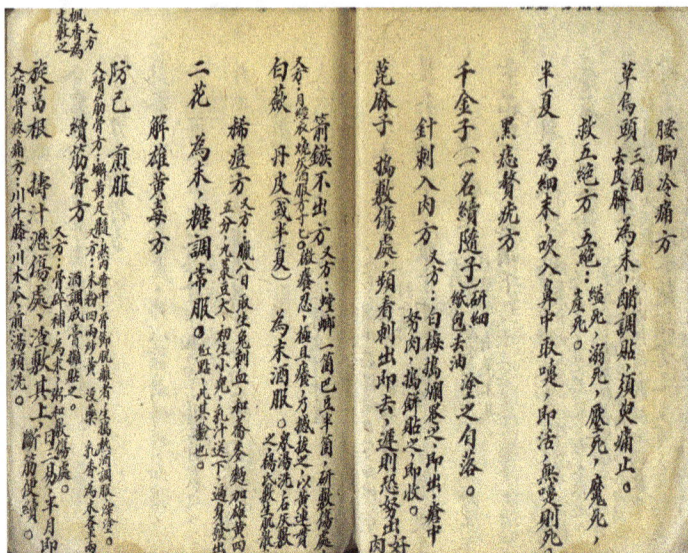

SURVEY OF CONTENTS: This volume is entirely devoted to 201 pharmaceutical recipes, including some with an approach of exorcism. Quite a few are focussed on curing poisoning resulting from opium smoking. The sequence of the recipes follows no apparent order. Most of the recipes have numerous ingredients. A few are single component recipes. The therapeutic indications are illnesses regularly encountered in rural regions, such as poisonous snake bites, rabid dog bites, injuries from falls and blows, conditions of "wind and warmth", sprained lower back and pain while breathing, lower back and legs feeling cold and pain, a needle having disappeared in the tissue, food poisoning, fish bones stuck in the throat, and also emergency treatments for acute diseases, and persons having attempted suicide.

\*\*\*

TITLE: (*Fu zhou za chao* 符咒雜抄, Copy of miscellaneous charms and spells)
ID: 8885
CONTENTS: Charms and spells
APPEARANCE: Simple ancient manuscript volume. Cover destroyed. Remaining parts covered with randomly scribbled characters, unrelated to the contents of this volume. Average calligraphy.

BINDING: Paper spills
MEASURE: 24.0 x 13.0
TITLE PAGE: No
NO. OF PAGES: 10
L.P. /CH.L: 8 x 24
LAYOUT: No lines, no frames
AUTHOR AND YEAR OF TEXT:
　　　　　　　Ancient but unidentifiable.
YEAR OF COPY: Possibly end of Qing dynasty, or Republican era.

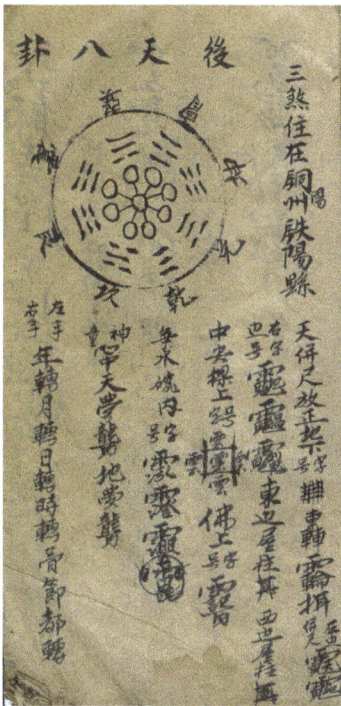

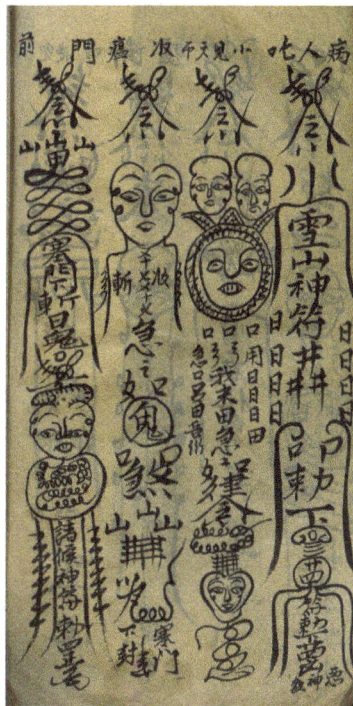

SURVEY OF CONTENTS: This is a manual on charms and spells. It is not an exorcistic book with a focus on curing illness. Rather, it happens to include illness therapy among other tasks performed by a Daoist practitioner. The text begins with a spell to stop bleeding: 斷血（至）〔止〕血用，口受. The following charms and spells follow no apparent sequence, structure, and focus: Ci zi qian tu sha yong zhu 此字千土煞用咒, "These characters can be used as a spell for thousands of local goblins". Hou tian ba gua 後天八卦, "Eight trigrams for [existence under] the latter heaven", 5 charms of different types to drive away evil, *jie yan* 解魘 "to dissolve nightmares", with 38 charms. Among the therapeutic indications of charms to be used for health care are *wen yi* 瘟疫, "warmth epidemics", *xiao er ye ti* 小兒夜啼, "children crying during the night", and *dian zi* 癲子, "peak-illness", i.e., psychiatric disorders.

*\*\**

| | |
|---|---|
| TITLE: | *Tian wen mi zhi* 天文秘旨, Secret messages hidden in the signs in heaven |
| ID: | 8886 |
| CONTENTS: | Daoism |
| APPEARANCE: | Ancient manuscript volume. Cover made from various layers of locally produced paper mulberry paper. It states no title. Careful copy. Calligraphy above average. |
| BINDING: | Thread |
| MEASURE: | 17.0 x 12.2 |
| TITLE PAGE: | No |
| NO. OF PAGES: | 28 |
| L.P. /CH.L: | 9 x 16 |
| LAYOUT: | No lines, no frames |

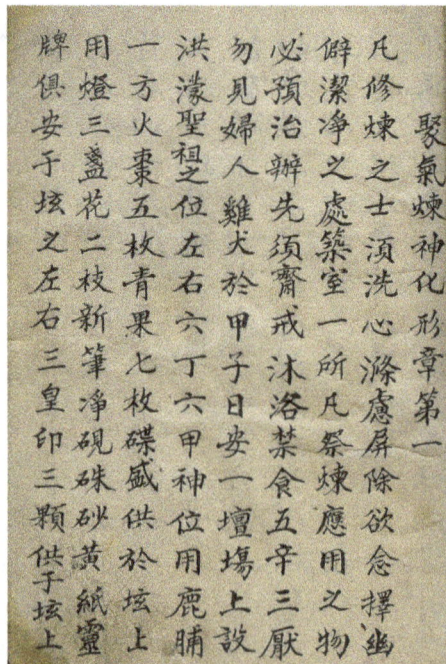

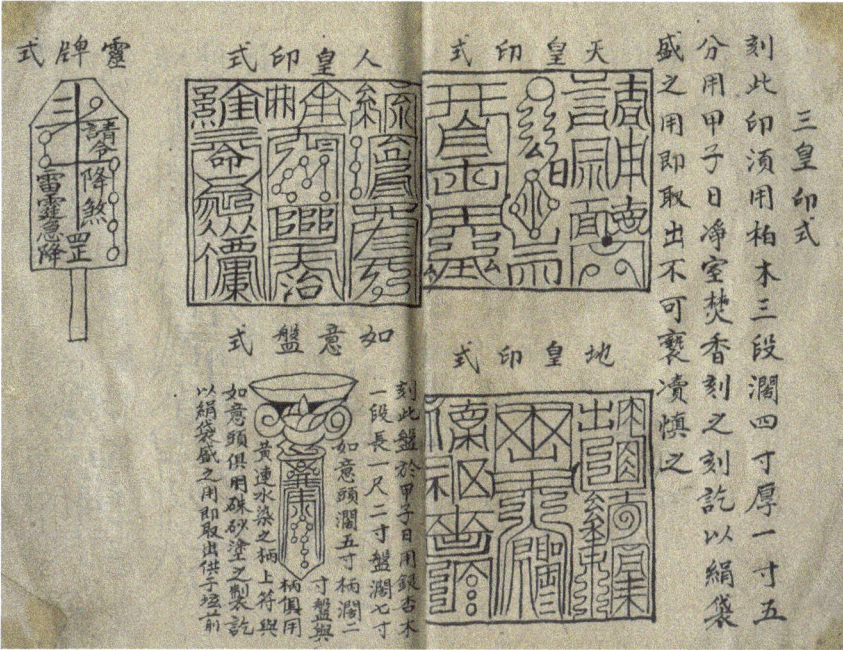

AUTHOR AND YEAR OF TEXT:     Unknown

YEAR OF COPY:    No Qing dynasty taboos observed. Republican era.

SURVEY OF CONTENTS: This is a Daoist manual. The text begins with Tian shu yuan shu 天書原序. "Celestial Writing. Original Preface." It is signed and dated as 軒轅二十三年......李百陽序. Next is Wan fa bao lu 萬法寶錄, "Precious Record of a Myriad Patterns," signed and dated as 龍明三年......通真子莊周謹序. One statement in this second preface reads: 予有洪鈞所授神書三卷，其一曰天文秘旨，其二曰天機玉函，其三曰道緣金鏡, "I have in my possession a divine text of three *juan* received from Hong Jun. The first is named 'Secret messages hidden in the signs of heaven'. The second is named 'The dynamics of heaven in a jade box' The third is named 'Golden Mirror of Dao and Fate'."

The main text begins with a Tian wen mi zhi. Mu lu 天文秘旨目錄, "Secret messages hidden in the signs in heaven. Table of contents," listing 9 sections:

聚氣鍊神化形　　第一、
太上飛昇印　　　第二、
斬三尸神　　　　第三、
周天吐納神術　　第四、
九轉金液丹　　　第五、
陰陽二氣丹　　　第六、

五氣朝元丹　　　第七、
八寶少陽丹　　　第八、
無極贊育丹　　　第九.

Apparently, this book is on the technique of refining one's body by means of breathing, lit.: "spitting and ingesting", *tu na* 吐納. However, the text also includes rituals, written charms and oral spells, such as 聚神符、鍊神符、化形符, pharmaceutical recipes, and also models for writing charms devoted to "the three august ones", *san huang yin shi* 三皇印式, i.e., *tian huang*, "the august one of heaven"; *di huang*, "the august one of the earth"; and *ren huang*, "the august one of man". Twelve drawings of *tai shang fei sheng yin shi* 太上飛昇印式, "Models for seals of Tai shan for flying and rising up in the air" further explain the aim of the refinement, that is an ability to fly and rise in the air. Only the section Zhou tian tu na shen shu 周天吐納神術, "The divine art of the universe's spitting and ingesting" resembles the technique of fetal breathing. All the other sections suggest an application of charms and other methods associated with Daoist elixir alchemy.

The *Tian wen mi zhi* 天文秘旨 is available as a regularly printed book.

*\*\**

| | |
|---|---|
| TITLE: | (*Yong ju ning chuang zhu* 癰疽疔瘡圖註, Comments on and illustrations of obstruction-illness and impediment-illness, pin-illness, and sores) |
| ID: | 8887 |
| CONTENTS: | External medicine |
| APPEARANCE: | Ancient manuscript volume. Paper aged, and with insect damage. Cover partly destroyed. No label with title or inscription. Average calligraphy. |
| BINDING: | Thread |
| MEASURE: | 23.5 x 12.8 |
| TITLE PAGE: | No |
| NO. OF PAGES: | 54 |
| L.P. /CH.L: | 8 x approx. 21 |
| LAYOUT: | No lines, no frames |
| AUTHOR AND YEAR OF TEXT: | |
| | Anonymous, Qing dynasty |
| YEAR OF COPY: | No Qing dynasty taboos observed. Republican era. |

SURVEY OF CONTENTS: This is a text from the realm of external medicine with a focus on *yong* 癰 and *ju* 疽 illnesses. The contents of this volume are very similar to those in ms. 8843. Both have drawings showing the location and names of *yong* 癰, "obstruction-illnesses", and *ju* 疽, "impediment-illnesses", with the following text offering explanations and advice on the preparation of pharmaceutical recipes. The drawings in the present volume lack individual headings.

A comparison with ms. 8843 shows that the very first drawing in the present volume constitutes the illustration Zheng mian shi er zheng tu 正面十二症圖, "Frontal view on 12 conditions", referred to in that volume, and showing the conditions 頂癰、螻蛄上串、螻蛄中串、螻蛄下串、痔漏, etc. The second drawing of the present volume shows a human figurine's back with names and locations of six conditions: 窄腮毒可敷、上發背、中發背、下發背、腎腰癰、騎馬癰不可敷. This drawing is not seen in ms. 8843. The 3rd drawing of the present volume resembles the drawing with the heading 側形十一症圖 in vol. 2 of ms. 8843. However, here the number of conditions shown is expanded to 15: 眉風毒、耳門癰、耳根癰、腮癰、中發疽、手發背、大腰帶、肘后癰、肘發疽、刺毒、腿癰、臍癰、裡廉、腳發背、外臁瘡. The fourth drawing is a view on a human figurine's back again, resembling the drawing with the heading 伏形十症圖 in ms. 8843. The conditions shown include 腦癰、鶴頂、三毒全、對口癰、肩癰、上搭背、中搭背、下搭背、天蛇頭、腰癰、委中毒. The fifth drawing shows a human figurine from its side. It lists 13 conditions: 鬢疽、瘰（痘）〔疽〕、面風疔、結喉癰、項癰、上肋疽、下肋疽、腎疽、凡刺毒又色蓮花、貼骨癰、腿游風、外廉、外拐. The sixth drawing is a frontal view; it resembles the drawing with the heading 正形十三症圖 in the second volume of ms. 8843. The conditions shown are 上眼丹、下眼丹、白面疔、鬚鬢、鬢毒、臂面毒、胳肢毒、乳毒、手膝、手心毒不可治、魚口、左右便毒、鶴膝風、膝腿毒、腳跟癰. The seventh drawing is another frontal view, showing nine conditions: 粉瘤、粉瘤、筋瘤可治、血瘤不可治、血瘤不可治、乳瘤不可治、發疽、脅毒、腿毒. Finally, the eighth drawing is a view from the side again, showing five conditions: 手疽、眉疽、耳疽、胲疽、赤白游風. These eight drawings are followed by more than 80 pharmaceutical recipes, most of them not from the realm of external medicine but from internal medicine and gynecology.

We have not been able to identify a printed text that may have been the source text of the present volume.

***

TITLE:　　　　*Ling ke fu ji* 灵科符集, Collection of charms from the numinous specialty [in medicine]

ID:　　　　　8888

CONTENTS:　 Daoist

APPEARANCE:     Ancient manuscript volume. Severe insect damage. Cover with inscription written with writing brush: 灵科符集. Average calligraphy.

BINDING:        Thread

MEASURE:        23.0 x 12.4

TITLE PAGE:     No

NO. OF PAGES:   12

L.P. /CH.L:     4-6 x 18

LAYOUT:         No lines, no frames

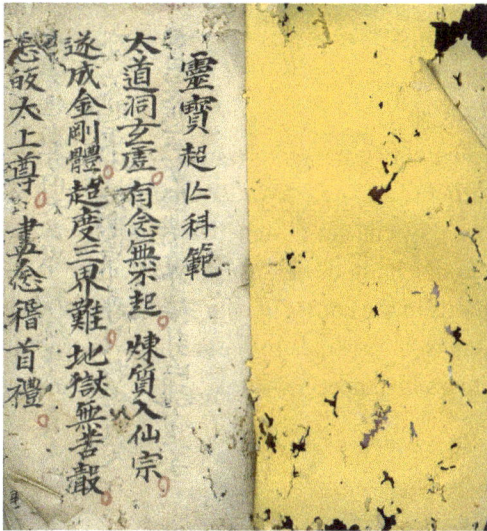

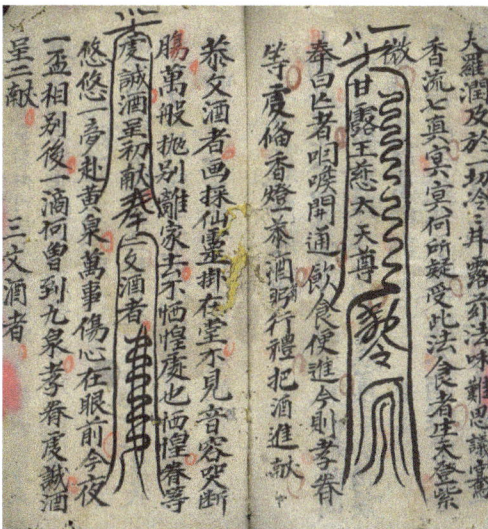

AUTHOR AND YEAR OF TEXT:
                    Unknown
YEAR OF COPY:     Character 玄 written to observe Qing dynasty taboo. Qing
                    dynasty.

SURVEY OF CONTENTS: This is a manual recording texts recited by Daoists to
expiate the soul of a deceased person. The very first section has the heading 靈
寶超亡科範. The text reads:
玉音仙範啓瑤臺，童子傳言地獄開。
爐炭鑊湯俱息冷，刀山劍柱化為塵。
真符告下羅酆去，地府迎將魂魄來。
讚詠一聲消萬罪，亡魂從此出泉台。
願薦此亡魂，往生神仙界.
Following this prologue two paragraphs are "Words to be spoken with rever-
ence", Bai gong wen 白恭文, and "Words to be spoken in prostration", Bai fu
wen 白伏文, followed by charms designed to attract a *hun* soul. There is also a
lengthy section, "to be chanted", 宜唱 *yi chang*, reciting the joys and sorrows,
partings and reunions in the course of a human life. There are further a chorus
and two charms, as well as rituals to be performed for guiding the soul of a
deceased person to a safe place.

***

TITLE:              *Qing xian li yi* 請仙禮儀, Etiquette to be observed when call-
                    ing on immortals
ID:                 8889
CONTENTS:       Daoist
APPEARANCE:     Ancient simple manuscript volume. No cover. Average cal-
                    ligraphy.
BINDING:         Paper spills
MEASURE:        16.7 x 14.2
TITLE PAGE:      No
NO. OF PAGES:    12
L.P. /CH.L:       8 x 13
LAYOUT:          No lines, no frames
AUTHOR AND YEAR OF TEXT:    Unknown
YEAR OF COPY:   No Qing dynasty taboos observed. Republican era.

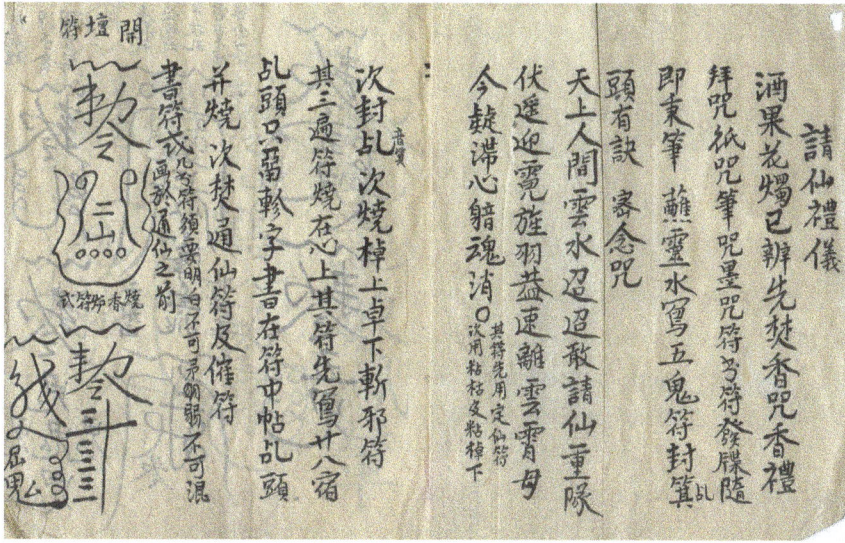

SURVEY OF CONTENTS: This is a Daoist manual. A heading on its first page states: Qing xian li yi 請仙禮儀, "Rituals associated with making requests to the immortals". The following text informs of details required in the performance of such rituals, including the use of items such as wine, fruit, ornamentary candles, and incense burning. This is followed by instructions on the type of paper, pen, and ink to be employed in writing the charms and written spells. The manuscript ends with a list of 108 charms of different styles

***

| | |
|---|---|
| TITLE: | *Yi fang zhai jin* 醫方摘錦, Brocade plucked from medical recipes. |
| ID: | 8890 |
| CONTENTS: | Pharmaceutical recipes |
| APPEARANCE: | Ancient manuscript volume. Margins and edges severely damaged. Written by various hands. Calligraphy in parts average, in parts clumsy. Cover |
| BINDING: | Thread |
| MEASURE: | 22.5 x 14.2 |
| TITLE PAGE: | Dirty. Inscription from left to right: 醫方摘錦/光緒叁拾叁年十壹月十九日立/俊生堂記 |
| NO. OF PAGES: | 19 |

L.P. /CH.L:        8 x 18
LAYOUT:            No lines, no frames
AUTHOR AND YEAR OF TEXT:
                   Anonymous, Qing dynasty
YEAR OF COPY:      No Qing dynasty taboos observed. Ink color relatively re-
                   cent. Republican era.

SURVEY OF CONTENTS: This is a casual record of pharmaceutical recipes and
items of related interest. It begins with 36 recipes recommended for treating
swelling and poison sores. This is followed by a section specifying the hierarchy
of nine echelons of social stratification *jiu liu* 九流: 一流舉子二流醫，三流風
水四流推，五流丹清六流畫，七僧八道九琴棋, "first echelon: scholars; sec-
ond echelon: physicians; third echelon, *feng shui* [practitioners]; fourth echelon: fortune tellers; fifth echelon: painters; sixth echelon: painters; seventh:
priests; eighth: Daoists; ninth: musicians."(The distinction between the two
types of painters categorized as occupying the fifth and sixth echelons is not
made clear.)

Next is a page with large characters combined from several individual characters. For example, the four characters 果老騎驢 are written to form one new composite character. Next is a paragraph on Ru shi dao san jiao 儒釋道三教, "The three teachings of Confucianism, Buddhism, and Daoism". These are rhetoric phrases used to attract customers for fortune telling. This is followed by a rhymed section with the title: Wai ke zheng zong yong ju zhu zheng ming shi 外科正宗癰疽諸症名十律, "Ten famous laws regarding all conditions of obstruction- and impediment-illness from the *Wai ke zheng zong*". It offers the names and the locations of different types of *yong* 癰 ("obstruction-illness") and *ju* 疽 ("impediment-illnesses"), i.e., specific types of abscesses believed to result from blockages in the pathways of qi.

The manuscript concludes with a listing of 26 pharmaceutical recipes for a broad variety of ailments including a "Wondrously effective recipe to strike the fetus," that is, for abortion, *da tai shen fang* 有打胎神方. The details are: *dou shuang* 豆双, one; *tai she xiang* 台射香, two *fen*; *ban mao* 班毛, three; *hong niang* 红娘, four; *shui zhi* 水蛭, one; *meng chong* 虻虫, three; *chuan jun* 川军, four *qian*. All ingredients are to be ground to a fine powder from which by means of honey are to be formed 3 pills. They are to be ingested with yellow wine. Another recipe has the name 飛燕迷春散, "Powder to make a flying swallow long for spring". It advises to prepare a powder from swallow fledglings and sprinkle it on a beautiful woman. This will make her willing to make love.

***

| | |
|---|---|
| TITLE: | *Tie da sun shang ling fu* 跌打損傷靈符, Magic charms for injuries from falls and blows. |
| ID: | 8891 |
| CONTENTS: | Charms and spells |
| APPEARANCE: | Ancient manuscript volume. Thin and simple. Average calligraphy. No cover. |
| BINDING: | Paper spills |
| MEASURE: | 16.7 x 14.3 |
| TITLE PAGE: | No |
| NO. OF PAGES: | 15 |
| L.P. /CH.L: | 8 x 14 |
| LAYOUT: | No lines, no frames |

AUTHOR AND YEAR OF TEXT:
    Unknown
YEAR OF COPY:   No Qing dynasty taboos observed. Republican era.

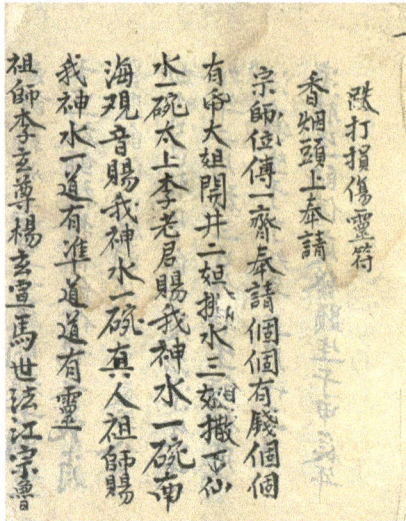

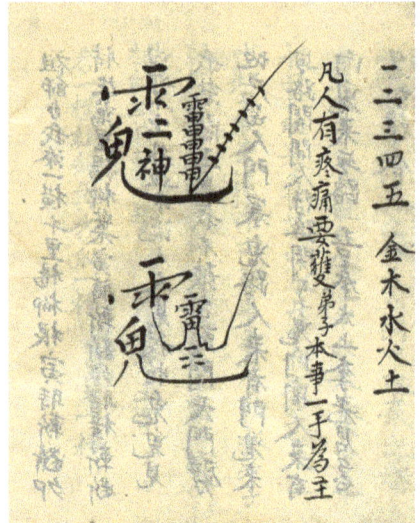

SURVEY OF CONTENTS: This is an exorcist's manual recording mostly simple and popular means to communicate with the spirits. A first part is a prayer to voice requests to the spirits. The spirits mentioned here are those familiar to the masses of the people. Examples are 王殷馬趙四大元帥、羅公師主，少時五郎列劉備、張飛并雲長，銅家子，鐵家郎，孫行者 (Sunxingzhe, the monkey known from the novel *Xi you ji* 西游记), 沙和尚 (Sha heshang, also known from the novel *Xi you ji* 西游记)，封刀接骨張九娘 (Zhang Jiuniang who gives a knife and sets fractures), and they are asked to *pi po pi xiang lian gu duan gu xiang jie* 皮破皮相連，骨斷骨相接, "When the skin is broken to make it connect again. When the bones are broken to join them again." Following this prayer 13 charms are drawn. Next is a prayer to be recited when sprinkling charm water, which is followed by five charms of the charm type, and then several charms with requests to spirits and to ward off demons. Further sections include a technique called *niao luan bi xing fa* 鳥卵弊形法, which is a "method to cause harm to one's physical body by means of a bird's egg", which is actually described as a technique, using the eggs of black chicken, to make one invisible. The following charms are recommended for "repelling weapons", *pi bing fu* 辟兵符, and for "keeping away disaster", *pi zai fu* 辟災 Next is a prayer to be recited when beheading a chicken, *zhan ji* 斬雞, and an advice on the meaning and use of a *lei yin* 雷印, "seal of the [Lord of] Thunder".

***

| | |
|---|---|
| TITLE: | *Yuan guang ming deng tong shu* 圓光明登通書, Halo brilliance almanac |
| ID: | 8892 |
| CONTENTS: | Daoist |
| APPEARANCE: | Ancient manuscript. Margins and edges damaged, but text complete. Cover dirty with inscription faintly readable: 道光拾年三月吉日立/惟口書. Average calligraphy. |
| BINDING: | Thread |
| MEASURE: | 18.8 x 14.0 |
| TITLE PAGE: | Inscription: 圓光明登通書全部 |
| NO. OF PAGES: | 44 |
| L.P. /CH.L: | 7 x 13 |
| LAYOUT: | No lines, no frames |
| AUTHOR AND YEAR OF TEXT: | |
| | Anonymous author. Qing dynasty. Copyist: Xu Guangneng 徐光瀧 |
| YEAR OF COPY: | Character 玄 not written to observe a Qing dynasty taboo. However, the reign period of *dao guang* 道光 is mentioned in the text. The present volume is an example of a text written during the Qing dynasty on a folk level where there was no concern over the observation of imperial taboos. Hence one can be certain that this volume was indeed written in the tenth year of the *dao guang* 道光 reign period, i.e., 1830. |

SURVEY OF CONTENTS: This is a manual of a folk exorcism practitioner. It begins with two prayers to the spirits. This is followed by a rarely seen explication of the sequence and meaning of individual strokes used in the writing of a charm. Subsequently, 13 charms are recorded for connecting with and voicing requests to the spirits. This is followed by an enumeration of utensils used for writing spells, and drawings of relevant charms. Next is a section Kai guang ke 開光科 with rather lengthy oral spells and simple charm drawings. A subsequent list of charms records different styles, including those of the composite

character type. At the end of this part of the volume an inscription says: 圓光
符書，徐光瀧記.

The second part of the volume is a different text with introductory headings on its first page: 靈符金書, 百水符, 大成金書　全部. Here the focus is on
exorcism for illnesses. The oral spells given and charms drawn here are recommended for twelve therapeutic indications, including *ya tong* 牙痛, tooth

ache, *bai bing* 百病, all types of diseases, *zhi xue* 止血, to stop bleeding, *xin teng* 心疼, heart/stomach pain, *wei qi tong* 胃氣痛, stomach qi pain; *wen yi* 瘟 疫, warmth epidemics, *zhi teng* 止疼, to end pain, *tou tong* 頭痛, headache, *yao teng* 藥疼, drug pain; *an tai* 安胎, to calm a fetus; *li ji* 痢疾, diarrhea; *cui sheng* 催生, to hasten birth; and *jie gu* 接骨, bonesetting. At the end of this second part an inscription says: 皇清道光十年三月十四日立神書.

***

TITLE:        (*Shang xue shou yao tu shi* 傷穴受藥圖式, Medication with illustrations for treating harm received at [insertion] holes)

ID:        8893

CONTENTS:        Bone setting – traumatology

APPEARANCE:        Ancient manuscript volume. Cover and beginning of text lost. Average calligraphy.

BINDING:        Thread

MEASURE:        19.6 x 12.2

TITLE PAGE:        No

NO. OF PAGES:        35

L.P. /CH.L:        8 x 21

LAYOUT:        No lines, no frames

AUTHOR AND YEAR OF TEXT:        Anonymous, Qing dynasty.

YEAR OF COPY:    No Qing taboo observed. Republican era.

SURVEY OF CONTENTS: This volume is a record of folk traumatology. It is special in that it offers drawings of human bodies showing the names and locations of "holes", *xue* 穴, a term usually reserved for acupuncture needle insertion points, and the effects of harm, exerted by "falls and blows", *tie da sun shang* 跌打損傷, received there. Each drawing is followed by a text recommending an appropriate treatment and providing the respective pharmaceutical recipes. The Berlin collections include several manuscript volumes with such an emphasis. However, they all differ in their contents. The headings of the drawings in the present volume are the following: 反背穴總圖、左相穴圖、右相穴圖、百會針圖、氣針左右側人穴法、氣針反背穴法總圖（以上均無解說文字）、左耳閉血、右耳大陰穴、對口穴、左右牙腮穴圖、咽喉穴圖、舌腌穴圖、頂圈鳳博穴、將臺血蒼穴、（乃傍）〔奶膀〕之左穴·二仙傳道圖、左血氣穴·右血爭穴圖、（乃棒）〔奶膀〕之下穴左右氣門之下圖、心頭中

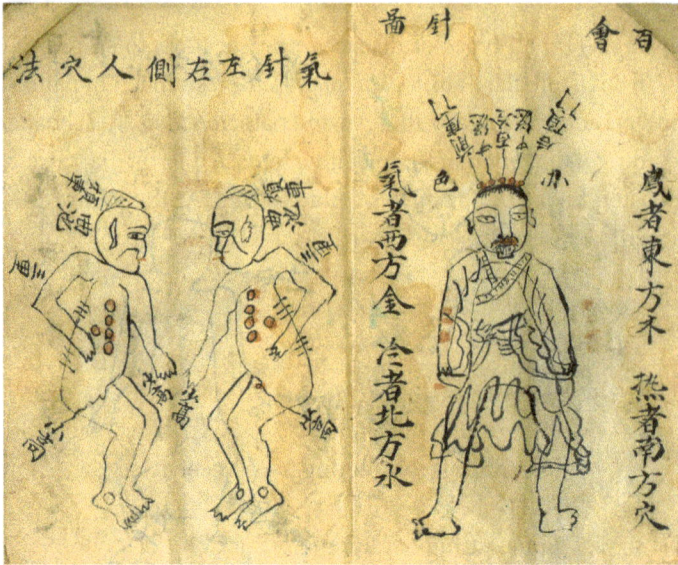

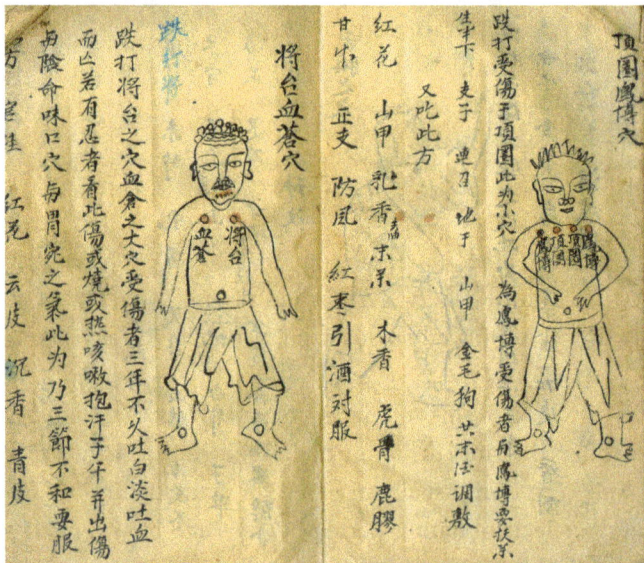

天針穴圖、心管穴圖、背偏人、鼻梁之穴圖、左淨（平）〔瓶〕·血腕穴圖、右血腕·淨（平）〔瓶〕穴圖、鳳翅盒弦穴、左邊骨穴圖、勾肚之血穴圖、鳳尾腰眼穴圖、左右兩脅雙掩穴圖、掛膀穴圖、腰中穴圖、銅壺滴漏穴圖、下喬穴圖、兩傍重骨之穴全圖、兩膊腕之全圖、背脊骨穴圖、兩腿穴圖、兩胃腕穴圖、肺經穴圖、掛下穴圖、胃宛骨穴圖、昏死在地全圖。

The pharmaceutical recipes provided include many simplifications and outright erroneous writings of the names of their ingredients, as for instance (the correct versions given in brackets): 然同（自然銅）、末藥（沒藥）、支

子（梔子）、地于（地榆）、玄乎（玄胡）、半下（半夏）、川夕（川牛膝）、只十（枳實）、子何車（紫河車）、兵卩（檳榔）、子中（紫草）、血結（血竭）、尔香（乳香）、一金·乙今（鬱金）、地別（地鱉）、碎甫（骨碎補）、宅南（澤蘭）、双生（桑寄生）、吉更（桔梗）、秦交（秦艽）. Quite a few of the substances used in the recipes are limited to folk use, as for instance: 矮腳傘、地南蛇、節骨丹、八龍麻、尋骨風、虎刺、活血丹.

\*\*\*

| | |
|---|---|
| TITLE: | (*Yao fang ji chao* 藥方集抄, Copy of a collection of pharmaceutical recipes) |
| ID: | 8894 |
| CONTENTS: | Pharmaceutical recipes |
| APPEARANCE: | Ancient manuscript volume. Margins and edges with some damage. Inferior calligraphy. |
| BINDING: | Thread |
| MEASURE: | 18.5 x 12.7 |
| TITLE PAGE: | No |
| NO. OF PAGES: | 39 |

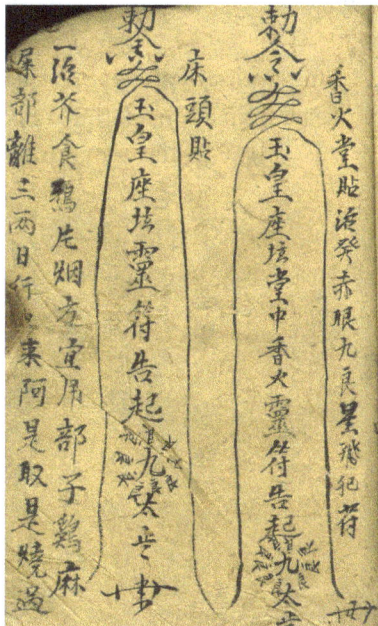

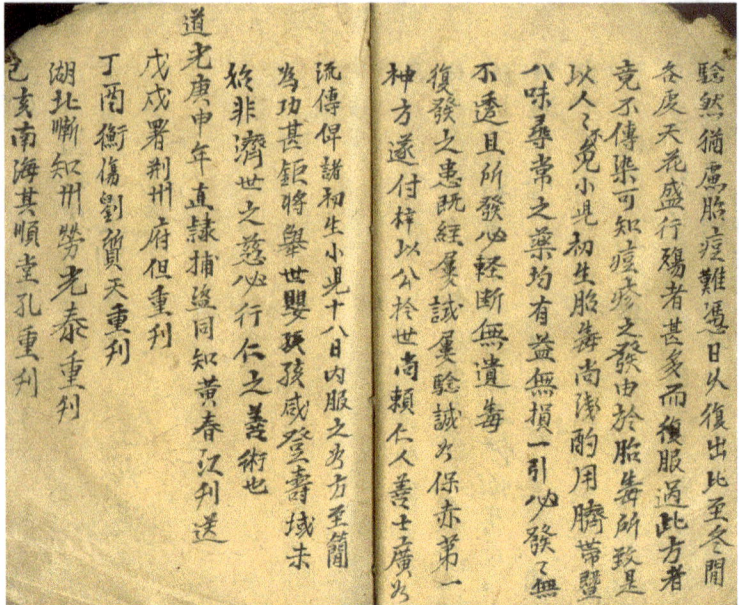

L.P. /CH.L:     8 x 17

LAYOUT:     No lines, no frames

AUTHOR AND YEAR OF TEXT:    Anonymous, Qing dynasty.

YEAR OF COPY:    The text mentions a year *geng shen* 庚申 of the *dao guang* 道光 reign period of the Qing dynasty (1840).

SURVEY OF CONTENTS: This is a list of 95 pharmaceutical recipes. The individual recipes were not copied from a single printed book, and there are only very few that appear to have originated from oral transmission. Most of the recipes were copied from diverse sources, including printed books and public announcements. The range of therapeutic indications is very broad, mostly from the specialties of gynecology, external medicine, pediatrics, and opthalmology. There is also a small number of apotropaic therapies.

\*\*\*

TITLE:    *Yao shu cheng fang* 藥書成方, Set recipes from materia medica books

ID:    8895

CONTENTS:    Pharmaceutical recipes

APPEARANCE:      Simple, crude ancient manuscript volume. Inferior calligraphy.

BINDING:      Paper spills

MEASURE:      19.4 x 14.1

TITLE PAGE:      Damaged with sections destroyed and missing. Remaining inscription: 藥書成方/□□□年□弍年巧月廿日吉旦/寶廿堂已記字十二張

NO. OF PAGES:      12

L.P. /CH.L:      6-9 x 19

LAYOUT:      No lines, no frames

AUTHOR AND YEAR OF TEXT:

      Unknown

YEAR OF COPY:      Republican era.

SURVEY OF CONTENTS: This is a listing of 35 pharmaceutical recipes, including three apotropaic approaches. The therapeutic indications include the following: 婦科補養 *fu ke bu yang*, "nourishment in gynecology"; 種子 *zhong zi*, "assisting fertility"; 乾血癆 *gan xue lao*, "dried blood exhaustion"; 吐血 *tu xue*, "blood-spitting"; 半身不遂 *ban shen bu sui*, "one half of the body paralyzed"; 乳汁不通 *ru zhi bu tong*, "milk flow blocked"; 乳癰 *ru yong*, "breast obstruc-

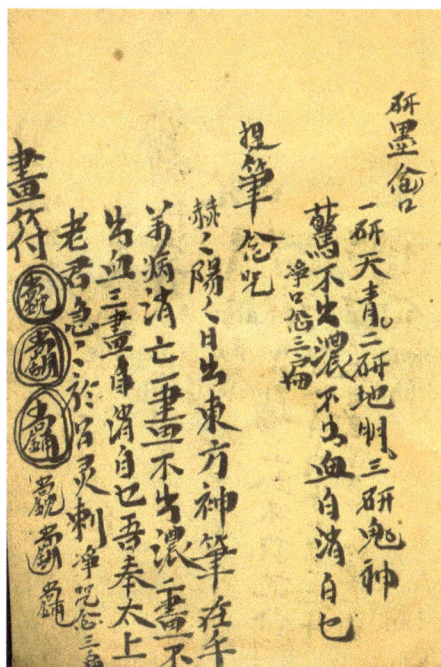

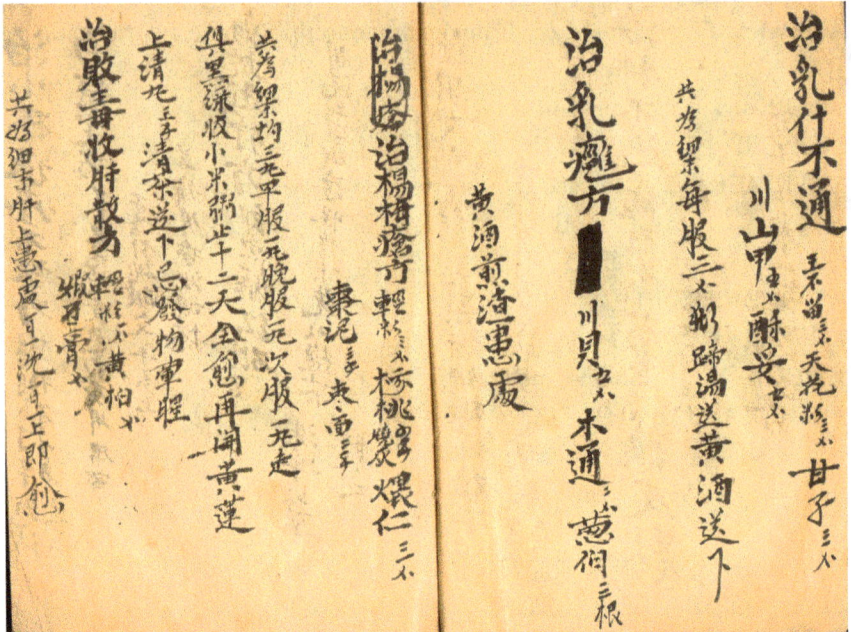

tion-illness"; 敗毒 *bai du*, "destructive poison"; 痘疹 *dou zhen*, "smallpox"; 疔瘡 *ding chuang*, "pin-illness sores"; 雜瘡 *za chuang*, "various sores"; 痢疾 *li ji*, "diarrhea"; 漏瘡 *lou chuang*, "seeping sores"; 瘟氣 *wen qi*, "warmth-illness qi"; 、眼疾 *yan ji*, "eye afflictions"; 下乳 *xia ru*, "to cause milk flow"; 黃水瘡 *huang shui chuang*, "yellow water sores"; 跌打損傷 *die da sun shang*, "injuries from falls and blows"; 腰腿疼 *yao tui teng*, "pain in the lumbar region and legs". There is one veterinary recipe. The majority of the recipes are fixed formulas as used in regular Chinese medicine. The list does not include purely orally transmitted single ingredient recipes.

The calligraphy and the scope of the illnesses to be treated suggest that this manuscript originates from the countryside, and was written by a person with a very low level of formal education. Nevertheless, the task was to record means to treat illnesses as conveniently as possible. The emphasis was on gynecological ailments and those associated with external medicine.

\*\*\*

TITLE:          *Shi liu lun tu shuo* 十六論圖說, Sixteen discourses, illustrated and discussed

ID:               8896

CONTENTS:        Smallpox

APPEARANCE:      Ancient manuscript volume. Cover with inscription written by later hand: 十六論圖說. Main text with exceptionally beautiful calligraphy. Careful handwriting. Accurate drawings.

BINDING:         Paper spills

MEASURE:         23.0 x 13.6

TITLE PAGE:      Two seals: Top ellipsoid: 昌邑县夏店区/黃家藥舖/東塚村. Below rectangular: 昌邑縣第一區第四十七保第十七甲圖記.

NO. OF PAGES:    17

L.P. /CH.L:      >7 x approx. 23

LAYOUT:          No lines, no frames

AUTHOR AND YEAR OF TEXT:

                 Unknown. Further research should determine whether this volume is related to the Yuan dynasty author Wei Junyong's 魏君用 (*Mi chuan*) *xiao er dou zhen jing yan liang fang* (秘传)小儿痘疹经验良方.

YEAR OF COPY:    No Qing dynasty taboos observed. Republican era.

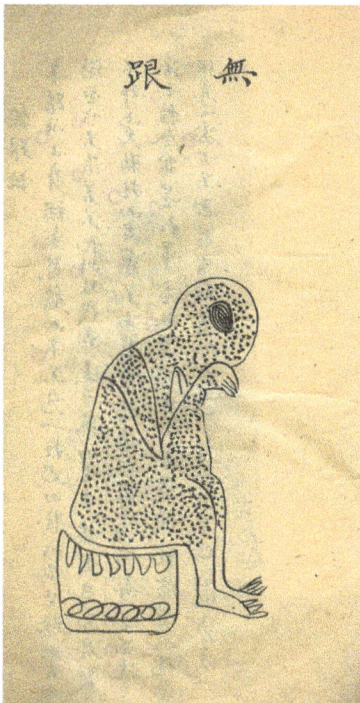

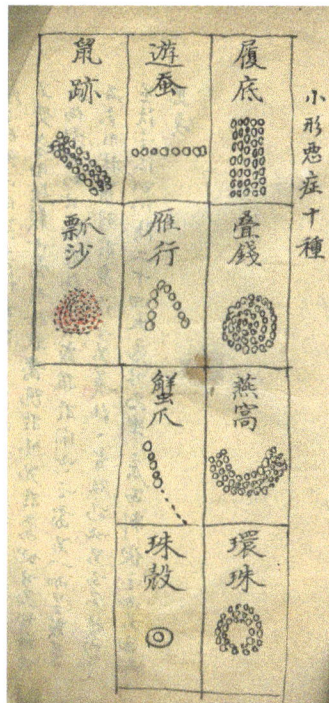

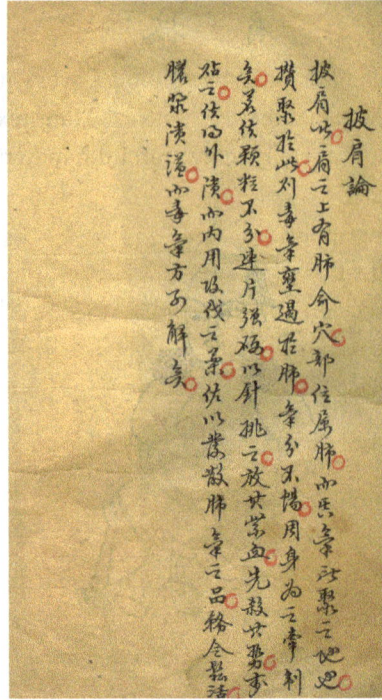

SURVEY OF CONTENTS: This volume focusses on smallpox. Its contents originate from the same printed book as those of ms. 8844: *Dou zhen jing yan liang fang* 痘疹經驗良方. Ms. 8844 has Er shi si tu zong lun 二十四圖總論, that is, "24 drawings of smallpox conditions with explanatory text". The present volume has 16 such conditions: 鎖項 鎖咽 披肩 攢胸 攢背 囊腹 纏腰 囊毬 鎖肛 鱗坐 抱膝 兩截 抱脛 無跟 四空 四實. It may well be that this volume has received a new binding after the initial eight sections were lost: 蒙頭 覆釜 抱鬢 蒙【骨丸】托腮 托頜 鎖口 鎖唇. Hence the title on the cover "16 Discourses and Drawings" represents the contents of the present fragment. A comparison with ms. 8844 shows further that the present volume does not include two sections 二十四圖治法總論 and 十圖治法總論, and it lacks the "Attached Recipes", 附方, present in the former. There is, however, in the present volume as in ms. 8844 a section 小形惡症十種. The drawings in the present volume are much finer than in ms. 8844, and they are colored.

\*\*\*

| | |
|---|---|
| TITLE: | *Xian guan you yi* 閑觀有益, To take time to view this will be beneficial |
| ID: | 8897 |
| CONTENTS: | Daoism |
| APPEARANCE: | Ancient manuscript volume with severe damage of the outer margins. |
| BINDING: | Paper spills |
| MEASURE: | 24.2 x 13.5 |
| TITLE PAGE: | Cover with inscription: 閑觀有益/王茂達記. Exquisite volume. Calligraphy and execution of drawings very delicate. |
| NO. OF PAGES: | 16 |
| L.P. /CH.L: | 6 x 25 |
| LAYOUT: | No lines, no frames |

AUTHOR AND YEAR OF TEXT:

Unknown. Comments by a Hu Zhuofeng 胡卓峰. Copied by Wang Maoda 王茂達

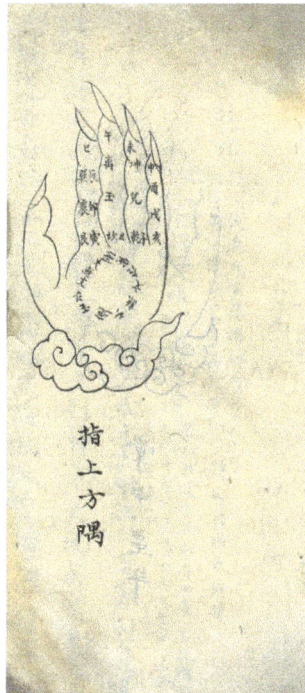

YEAR OF COPY:    Qing dynasty taboos observed throughout. Character 玄
                 written with final stroke omitted. Date provided at the end
                 of the text: 大清光緒捌年菊月重陽日抄. Hence the volume
                 was prepared in 1882.

SURVEY OF CONTENTS: This is a Daoist text. The first page shows a very del-
icately executed Shen zhong zao hua zhi tu 身中造化之圖. This is a simpli-
fied version of the Daoist *Nei jing tu* 內景圖. It is followed by an explanatory
text the title of which is only partly readable: 造化圖（說?）. A key sentence
states: 夫人亦一小天也盖神中一窍一节莫不有神居焉, "Now, man is a small
heaven too. The fact is, in each orifice, in each joint in the human body resides
a spirit". This is followed by a text Zhuofeng Hu xian sheng zu qi bei jiao zhi lun
卓峰胡先生祖炁被繳直論, "Straightforward discourse by Mr. Hu Zhuofeng on
the reception of ancestral qi", a basic statement from the realm of *qi gong* 氣
功 of that time. Next are several brief paragraphs devoted to the acquisition
of various types of qi, including 祖炁詳論, 取祖炁法, 論取罡訣, 取魁炁法, 取
煞炁法, 取生炁法, 取火炁法, 取金光法, 取水炁法. They all are related to the
techniques of refining qi. The volume ends with two delicate drawings of stel-
lar constellations projected onto the palm and inner side of the fingers, as well
as several pages under the heading San dong zhai fa 三洞齋法, with explica-
tions of Daoist rituals.

***

TITLE:            *Zhen mai yao jue* 診脈要訣, Essential instructions on vessel
                  diagnosis.
ID:               8898
CONTENTS:         Vessel diagnosis
APPEARANCE:       Ancient manuscript volume. Original cover lost. Kraft paper
                  cover added by later hand. Inscription with fountain pen: 診
                  脈要訣目錄. Handwriting and calligraphy above average.
BINDING:          Thread
MEASURE:          20.0 x 13.0
TITLE PAGE:       No
NO. OF PAGES:     34
L.P. /CH.L:       13 x 28
LAYOUT:           No lines, no frames

AUTHOR AND YEAR OF TEXT:

Chen Wenzhi 陳文治, Ming dynasty

YEAR OF COPY: Qing dynasty taboos observed throughout. Character 玄 written with final stroke omitted. Character 寧 written in abbreviated version. End of Qing dynasty.

SURVEY OF CONTENTS: This manuscript volume is focussed on vessel diagnosis. The text is preceded by three explanatory lines: 診脈要訣/秀水鶴溪陳文治輯/門人醫官劉得懋校. The volume begins with a table of contents; the main text begins with a "Rhyme on defining the positions of *cun, guan, chi*", Cun guan chi ding wei ge 寸關尺定位歌, followed by an "illustration of the positions and physical appearance of the vessels of both hands", 兩手脈位形圖 liang shou mai wei xing tu, and the sections 臟腑定位歌, 總脈名歌, 七表脈形歌, 八裏脈形歌, 九道脈形歌, 長短牢疾大小脈形歌, 脈形圖說. The section "Drawings and discussion of different shapes of vessel [movements]" lists 30 illustrations of pulses, and states: 本靜齋圖註及宗叔和脈經，輯略於此. That is, this section is based on the Ming author Zhang Shixian's 張世賢 (Tiancheng 天成, Jingzhai 靜齋) *Tu zhu nan jing mai jue* 圖註難經脈訣. A comparison of the contents of the present volume with that book shows that four sections 鬼賊脈歌, 四時虛實脈歌, 足三脈歌, 形證色脈應否歌 are missing here.

Chen Wenzhi 陳文治 lived during the *wan li* 萬曆 and *chong zhen* 崇禎 reign periods. Of his writings the *Guang si quan jue* 廣嗣全訣, 12 *juan*; *Yang ke xuan cui* 瘍科選粹, 8 *juan*; *Zhu zheng ti wang* 諸證提綱, 10 *juan*; and the *Shang han ji yan* 傷寒集驗, 6 *juan*, still exist. The present text is not listed in the *Zhong guo zhong yi gu ji zong mu* 中國中醫古籍總目; it appears to have been lost. Hence this manuscript volume is of extraordinary research value, even though it is only a fragment.

***

| | |
|---|---|
| TITLE: | *Shang han bing zheng tan tou* 傷寒病證湯頭, Decoction recipes for disease signs of harm caused by cold |
| ID: | 8899 |
| CONTENTS: | Harm caused by cold |
| APPEARANCE: | Ancient manuscript volume. Cover faintly greenish-blue. Inside paper color aged. Cover with inscription, upper left: 傷寒病證湯頭. Below this title, personal seal with four characters: 文奇克印. Title and contents do not agree. Careful handwriting. Good calligraphy. |
| BINDING: | Thread |
| MEASURE: | 23.0 x 13.5 |
| TITLE PAGE: | No |

NO. OF PAGES:    35

L.P. /CH.L:    8 x 20

LAYOUT:    No lines, no frames

AUTHOR AND YEAR OF TEXT:

    Anonymous, Qing dynasty.

YEAR OF COPY:    Character 玄 written with final stroke omitted. Character 寧 written in abbreviated version. Qing dynasty, *dao guang* 道光 reign period or thereafter.

SURVEY OF CONTENTS: The contents of this volume are mostly written in rhymes. However, the topics treated are heterogenous. They are entirely un-related to the health issues of "harm caused by cold" referred to in the title on the cover. At this moment we are not in a position to determine whether this volume is a copy of a printed book, or whether the writer himself composed all the rhymed paragraphs. To facilitate later investigations into the origins of its contents, the headings of the sections are listed here in full, with explanatory notes in brackets:

經產六合湯、婦人胎前禁忌藥、喉方、傷寒脈歌兼傷風 (These three paragraphs are rhymes with seven-characters lines)、四診脈訣 (four-charac-ters per line. A comparison with the *Cui zhen ren mai jue* 崔真人脈訣 and the *Si yan ju yao* 四言舉要 has found no parallels. This is a different poem)、浮沉遲數四脈 (not rhymed)、七表八里總歸四脈 (seven characters per line)、

內因脈、外因脈、不內不外因脈、定死脈形候歌、太陽風邪傷衛脈證、太
陽寒邪傷營脈證、風寒營衛同病脈證、三陽受病傳經訣慾癒脈證、陽明表
病脈證、陽明熱病脈證、陽明府病脈證、陽明慎汗慎清慎下、少陽脈證、
少陽病用柴胡湯加減法、少陽禁汗禁吐禁下、少陽可汗可吐可下、三陽合
病并病、三陰受病傳經欲癒脈證、太陰陰邪脈證、太陰陽邪脈證、太陰陽
明表裡同病、少陰陰邪脈證、少陰陽邪脈證、少陰太陽表裡同病、厥陰陰
邪脈證、厥陰陽邪脈證、兩感、汗下失宜致變壞證、表證、里證、陽證、
陰證、陽盛格陰、陰盛格陽、陽毒、陰毒、表熱里熱陰熱陽熱、惡寒背寒
寒辨、惡風、頭痛、項強、身痛、煩躁不眠懊憹、自汗頭汗、手足汗、潮
熱時熱、譫語鄭聲、渴證、舌胎、胸脅滿痛、嘔證、往來寒熱如瘧寒熱、
腹滿痛、吐證、熱利寒利、但欲寐、陰陽咽痛、氣上衝、飢不欲食、手足
厥逆、少腹滿痛、神昏狂亂蓄血發狂、循衣摸床、太陽陽邪停飲、太陽陰
邪停飲、少陰陽邪停飲、少陰陰邪停飲、喘息短氣、心下悸、戰振慄、呃
逆噦噫、結胸、痞鞕（鞭）、發黃、疹斑、衄血、吐血、大小便膿血、頤
毒、狐惑、百合、熱入血室、食復勞復、房勞復陰陽易.

***

| | |
|---|---|
| TITLE: | (*Hou ke san shi liu zheng* 喉科三十六症, Thirty six pathological conditions in laryngology) |
| ID: | 8900 |
| CONTENTS: | Laryngology |
| APPEARANCE: | Ancient manuscript volume. Cover added by later hand. Inscription: 咽喉論. Below, personal seal, round: 文【大口？】克印. Average calligraphy. |
| BINDING: | Thread |
| MEASURE: | 20.1 x 13.2 |
| TITLE PAGE: | No |
| NO. OF PAGES: | 64 |
| L.P. /CH.L: | 7 x approx. 16 |
| LAYOUT: | No lines, no frames |
| AUTHOR AND YEAR OF TEXT: | |
| | Unknown |
| YEAR OF COPY: | The character 玄 is not written with the final stroke omitted. Republican era. |

SURVEY OF CONTENTS: This is a book on laryngology. Its title, *Yan hou lun* 咽喉論 is listed twice in the *Zhong guo zhong yi gu ji zong mu* 中國中醫古籍總目; once as a book compiled by the Qing author Lu Nanxuan 逯南軒, with a first edition published in 1783, and second as an anonymous manuscript volume with two appendices: Mi shou hou ke 秘授喉科, "Secretly transmitted laryngology", and Yan ke yuan shi xin yao 眼科原始心要, "The essence of ophthalmology, personal experience". Whether the present volume is related to one or both of these books remains to be examined.

The names of illness affecting the throat listed in the present volume, as well as the style of its drawings, in many respects parallel those documented in ms. 8930. The drawings always show a circle with a section *di ding* 帝丁, representing the uvula, in the middle at the top. In some of the circles, on the left and right the tonsils are drawn, and in the center the tip of the tongue. To facilitate

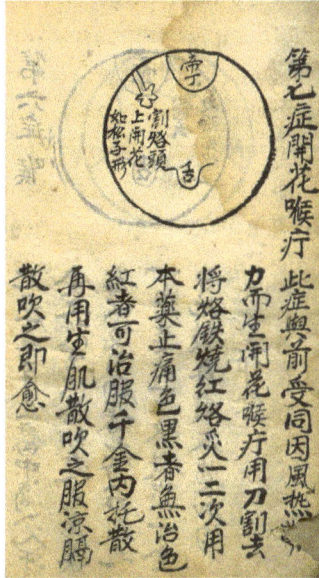

later comparative research, all 36 conditions recorded and illustrated in the present volumes are listed here as follows:

第一症纏喉風、第二症慢喉風、第三症鎖〔喉〕風、第四症雙乳蛾、第五症單乳蛾、第六症喉、第七症開花喉疔、第八症喉疳瘡、第九症雙喉癰、第十症蓮花毒、第十一症【口秦】舌〔瘡〕、第十二症右雀舌、第十三症左雀舌、第十四症纏舌風、第十五症走馬喉風、第十六症走馬疳、第十七症死雙乳蛾核、第十八症活雙乳蛾核、第十九症氣丹、第二十症喉痹、第廿一症匝舌癰、第廿二症小兒舌下珍珠、第廿三症小兒上顎、第

廿四症舌上紅癰、第廿五症吹舌喉風、第廿六症左右死乳、第廿七症回食
丹、第廿八症兜腮癰、第廿九症重舌癰、第卅症舌上生瘡、第卅一症舌上
癰、第卅二症兩腮熏黑、第卅三症舌上死癰、第卅四症出汗生癰、第卅五
症左陽瘡、第卅六症右陰瘡.

Following these 36 conditions is a list of 71 pharmaceutical recipes, mostly
with therapeutic indications from the realm of laryngology, including advice
on their special pharmaceutical preparation. The recipes include quotes from
the *Cheng Xinghai yi an* 程星海醫案, a rarely seen book published at the end of
the Ming dynasty, around 1621, by Cheng Lun 程崙, Xinghai 星海.

The section following the recipes has the heading Hou ke lun 喉科論, "On
laryngology". This is a discourse on the diagnosis and therapies of all types of
throat diseases. It parallels in many respects a lengthy attachment in the final
section of ms. 8830. Presumably ms. 8830 and the present volume originated
from the same source. The therapies emphasized in the present volume include pharmaceutical treatment, needling, as well as anesthesia and surgery.
Such a variety of therapeutic approaches is rarely documented in comparable
books on laryngology. Their sources remain to be determined.

The volume concludes with a section with the title Mai jue 脈訣, "Instructions on vessel [movements]", a list of pharmaceutical drugs assumed to guide
others into specific conduits, a list of pharmaceutical drugs with adverse syn-
ergisms, and a discourse on ulcers and abscesses.

***

| | |
|---|---|
| TITLE: | *Qing shen yi zong* 請神一宗, A lineage of calling on the gods |
| ID: | 8901 |
| CONTENTS: | Exorcism |
| APPEARANCE: | 2 ancient manuscript vols. Paper turned yellow-brown from smoke. Margins with some damage; text complete. Careful handwriting. Average calligraphy. Cover and text on iden- tical paper. One volume with recent ballpoint pen inscrip- tion: 鬼咒神符之宝. Second volume with date on last page: 加慶廿三年正月吉良親填符書弟子續道法無邊 |
| BINDING: | Thread |
| MEASURE: | 20.6 x 11.0 |
| TITLE PAGE: | No |

NO. OF PAGES: Vol. 1: 25. Vol. 2: 38
L.P. /CH.L: Mostly 6 x approx. 22
LAYOUT: No lines, no frames

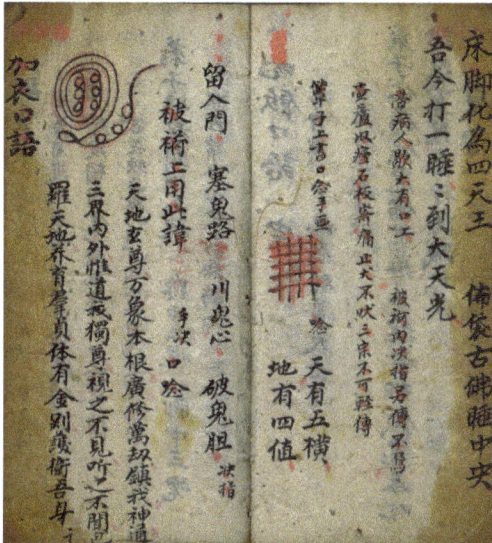

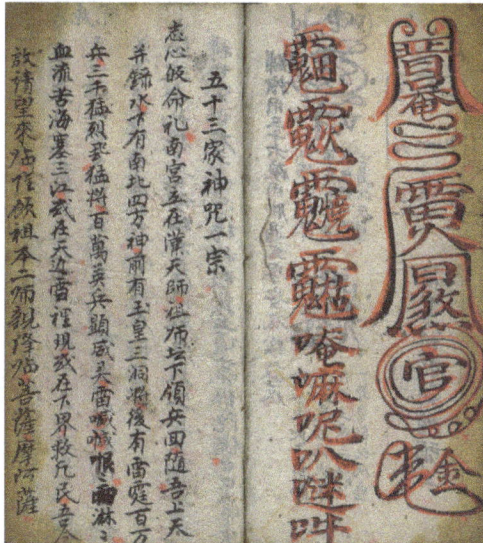

AUTHOR AND YEAR OF TEXT:
Anonymous, Qing dynasty.
YEAR OF COPY: Qing dynasty taboos not observed. Possibly Republican era.

SURVEY OF CONTENTS: These two volumes offer rich data on exorcism. Vol. 1 begins with a section Qing shen yi zong 請神一宗. These are 14 paragraphs with prayers asking all types of spirits for assistance. The spirits are mostly those of the Daoist pantheon. This is followed by patterns of prayers/orations advising believers how to address the spirits. Next is a section Qi shi yi zong 啓師一宗, that is, a request towards priests/monks to fulfill the requests of believers. A subsequent section Chi fan kou yü yi zong 吃飯口語一宗 and Ye su yi zong 夜宿一宗 are exorcistic spells to threaten malign demons, combining manual gestures and written charms. Next is a section Da fu yi zong 打符一宗, offering numerous written charms which have been redrawn with vermilion ink to increase their power. The charms cover the entire hight of a page.

Vol. 2 begins with a prayer to the founder of the school to ward off warmth epidemics. The section Da tao tang yi zong 打桃湯一宗 lists numerous different, often rarely seen charms. The sections Chan xian kou yu 纏線口語 and Dao jin kou shang 到禁口上 advise on manual exorcistic gestures. Not all of these rituals are designed to ward off disease. Some interdictions serve to end consumption of alcoholic beverages, and to stop the beating of gongs and drums.

The charms listed in this manuscript are very many, the accompanying incantations are very long, as well as refined and enigmatic.

***

| | |
|---|---|
| TITLE: | (*Yan ke jie chao* 眼科節抄. Copy of selected issues from ophthalmology) |
| ID: | 8902 |
| CONTENTS: | Ophthalmology |
| APPEARANCE: | Simple ancient manuscript volume. Dirty cover without title. Careful handwriting. Average calligraphy. |
| BINDING: | Thread |
| MEASURE: | 17.9 x 13.2 |
| TITLE PAGE: | No |
| NO. OF PAGES: | 12 |
| L.P. /CH.L: | 6-10 x 20 |
| LAYOUT: | No lines, no frames |
| AUTHOR AND YEAR OF TEXT: | |
| | Cheng Songya 程松崖; Ming dynasty. |
| YEAR OF COPY: | Paper quality and ink color suggest Republican era. |

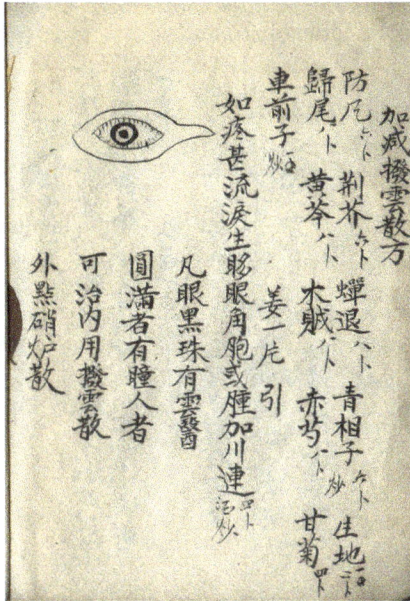

SURVEY OF CONTENTS: This volume focusses on the diagnosis and treatment of eye afflictions. It has neither preface nor postscript, or notes on the use of the book. The author remains unknown. The text comprises 17 identical illustrations of eyes without any hint at how they should relate to diagnosis and pharmaceutical therapy described in the accompanying paragraphs. The final section of the volume is a list of several pharmaceutical recipes for use in ophthalmology. Apparently, the copyist excerpted his data from the Ming author Cheng Songya's 程松崖 *Yan ke ying yan liang fang* 眼科应验良方.。

*** 

| | |
|---|---|
| TITLE: | *Xiao er ke tui ni* 小兒科推拿, Pediatric push-and-pull massage. |
| ID: | 8903 |
| CONTENTS: | Pediatrics |
| APPEARANCE: | Ancient manuscript volume. Rough, filthy cover with inscription: 小兒科推拿/李氏. Inferior calligraphy, but careful handwriting. |
| BINDING: | Paper spills with kraft paper cover wrapped and pasted around the back of the volume. |
| MEASURE: | 22.2 x 14.0 |

TITLE PAGE: No. No table of contents.
NO. OF PAGES: 23
L.P. /CH.L: 8 x approx. 21
LAYOUT: No lines, no frames
AUTHOR AND YEAR OF TEXT:
Xia Ding 夏鼎, Yuzhu 禹鑄. Qing dynasty.
YEAR OF COPY: No Qing dynasty taboos observed. Republican era.

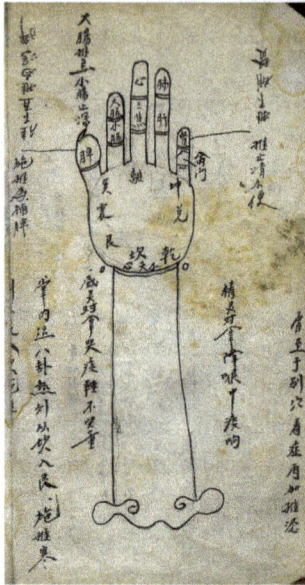

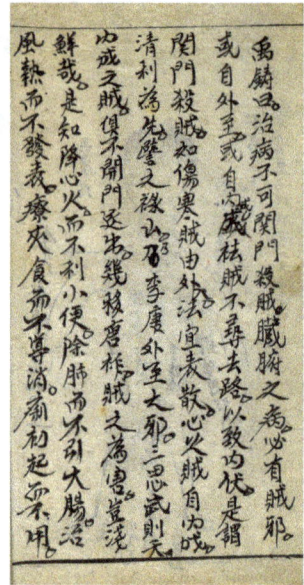

SURVEY OF CONTENTS: This is an illustrated text on *tuina* 推拿– push and pull massage. The first page shows a frontal view of a face indicating the locations of 百會穴, 囟門窩, and 太陽. Below the drawing is an explanatory text. On the following pages seven drawings of arms, legs, and the entire human body show the locations of relevant acupuncture needle insertion "holes", *xue* 穴. In the accompanying text one repeatedly encounters phrases like *Yu Zhu yue* 禹鑄曰, "Yuzhu stated", *Zhuoxi jia chuan kou jue* 卓溪家傳口訣, "Oral instructions passed on in the family of Zhuoxi", and *Tui na dai yao fu* 推拿代藥賦, "The replacement of pharmaceutical drugs by push-and-pull massage. A poem". Apparently, the present volume is a partial copy of the Qing author Xia Ding 夏鼎, Yuzhu's 禹鑄 *You ke tie jing* 幼科鐵鏡 of 1695.

\*\*\*

| | |
|---|---|
| TITLE: | *San shi liu she. Za fang quan tu* 三十六舌·雜方全圖. Thirty six tongues. Miscellaneous recipes, completely illustrated. |
| ID: | 8904 |
| CONTENTS: | Tongue diagnosis, pharmaceutical recipes |
| APPEARANCE: | Fine ancient manuscript volume. Brown-red cover. Calligraphy at times disorderly, at times careful. Some passages filled in by later hand. |
| BINDING: | Thread |
| MEASURE: | 23.1 x 12.5 |
| TITLE PAGE: | With inscription written by later owner, from left to right: 上卷三十六舌下卷雜方全圖/皇清道光廿貳年壬寅歲季冬月景城堂劉記/黃翼俊. Four square shaped seals with characters cut in relief, red: 劉金高記, and 榴金高記. Three oval seals, with illegible characters cut in relief, red. |
| NO. OF PAGES: | 31 |
| L.P. /CH.L: | 9 x approx. 24 |
| LAYOUT: | No lines, no frames |
| AUTHOR AND YEAR OF TEXT: | |
| | Liu Jingao 劉金高. Ca. 1842 to early Republican era. |

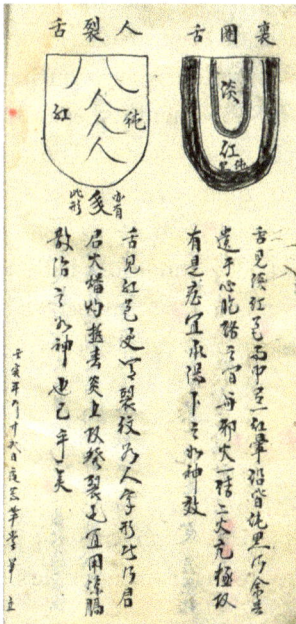

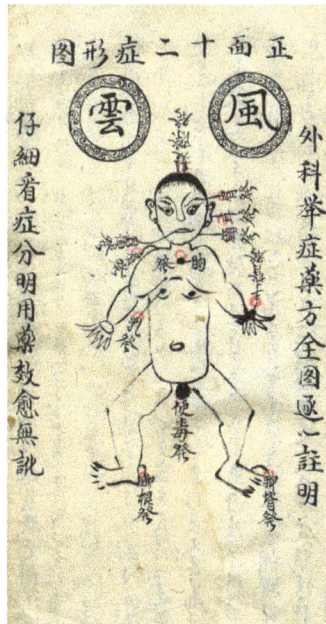

YEAR OF COPY:　　Date stated on title page: 1843. However, the quality of the paper and the failure to observe Qing dynasty taboos let this date appear questionable. Maybe it was added by a later hand.

SURVEY OF CONTENTS: This manuscript has two distinct parts. The first part has the title *Ao shi shang han jin jing lu* 敖氏傷寒金鏡錄, "Mr. Ao's golden mirror record of harm caused by cold"; it includes the drawings and explanations of 36 tongue appearances. It begins with a preface failing to specify its author, place, and time. This is followed by 36 drawings of tongues with different coatings covering the upper third of a page, and an explanatory text in the two lower thirds. The *Ao shi shang han jin jing lu* 敖氏傷寒金鏡錄 of 1341 was compiled by the Yuan author Du Ben 杜本 (*hao*: Qingbi 清碧). In the course of its transmission in subsequent centuries it was often modified. Hence it is rather difficult to determine exactly the original edition from which the contents of the present manuscript volume were copied. Following the list of 36 different tongue appearances is a list of more than 70 pharmaceutical recipes. These are mostly folk recipes relying on one single component.

　　The second part has the title *Wai ke ju zheng yao fang quan tu zhi yi zhu ming* 外科舉症藥方全圖逐一註明. "Explanatory notes on all conditions in external medicine with pharmaceutical recipes and a complete illustration". These are folk pharmaceutical recipes for external medicine in a frequently seen style. The structure is always such that a section begins with a drawing of a complete human body, and on this drawing the locations of certain ailments from the realm of external medicine are shown. Subsequently, these ailments are discussed in the text, with pharmaceutical recipes added. The present volume has only two such sections: Bei xing qi zheng tu shi 背形七症圖式, "Graphic illustration of seven conditions on the back", and Zheng mian shi er zheng xing tu 正面十二症形圖, "Illustration of twelve conditions with frontal view". They are followed by a list of numerous pharmaceutical recipes under the title Yi fang bian lan 醫方便覽, "A brief guide to medical recipes".

***

TITLE:　　　　　*Nan ji tian hua bao lu zhu you ke fu zhuan* 南極天華寶錄祝由科符篆, Precious record reflecting the south pole's celestial splendor in charm seals from the specialty of invocation of the origin

ID:              8905
CONTENTS:        Exorcism
APPEARANCE:      Ancient manuscript volume. Kraft paper cover. No title. Calligraphy above average.
BINDING:         Thread
MEASURE:         19.3 x 13.7
TITLE PAGE:      No. No table of contents.
NO. OF PAGES:    42
L.P. /CH.L:      11 x 24
LAYOUT:          No lines, no frames
AUTHOR AND YEAR OF TEXT:
                 Anonymous, Qing dynasty.
YEAR OF COPY:    Character 玄 not written to observe a Qing dynasty taboo. Republican era.

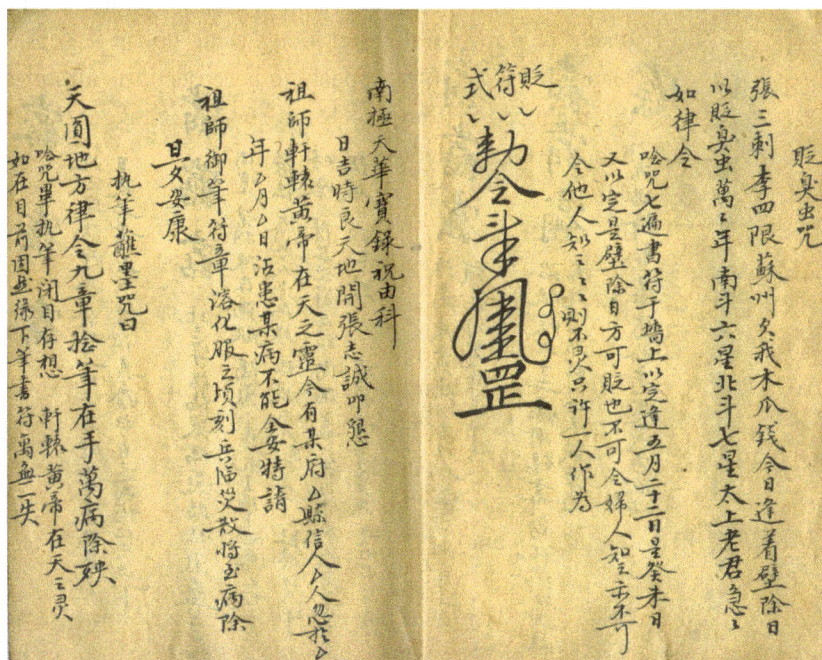

SURVEY OF CONTENTS: This is an exorcist's manual with various types of charms and their explanations. The first seven pages are devoted to charms made up of Chinese characters, mostly with the character 尚 as their heading.

Less often these charms have the character 食 or 雨 as their major constituting element. The main part of the book follows the title *Nan ji tian hua bao lu
zhu you ke fu zhuan* 南極天華寶錄祝由科符篆. Here the sequence of charms
is numbered from 1 to 126. Each charm is preceded by the name of a "celestial
physician", and is surrounded by one or two orations. The *Nan ji tian hua bao lu
zhu you ke fu zhuan* 南極天華寶錄祝由科符篆 is a widely available printed text
from the specialty of *zhu you ke* 祝由科. It needs not be described in detail here.

***

| | |
|---|---|
| TITLE: | *Wan fa gui zong* 萬法歸宗, A myriad patterns based in the ancestral lineage |
| ID: | 8906 |
| CONTENTS: | Exorcism |
| APPEARANCE: | Ancient manuscript volume. Margins and edges severely damaged. The cover was taken from another manuscript. Inside of front cover inscription upside down: 毛存良記. Mao Cunliang 毛存良 appears to have been the author of the manuscript from which the cover was taken. Careful handwriting but deficient calligraphy. |
| BINDING: | Thread |
| MEASURE: | 21.4 x 11.2 |
| TITLE PAGE: | No |
| NO. OF PAGES: | 40 |
| L.P. /CH.L: | Single line frame |
| LAYOUT: | Pages without charm drawings: 9 x approx. 16. Edges with upper side black fish tale. |
| AUTHOR AND YEAR OF TEXT: | |
| | Unknown |
| YEAR OF COPY: | Republican era. |

SURVEY OF CONTENTS: The *Wan fa gui zong* 萬法歸宗 is a well-known Daoist book; it was included in the *Xu xiu si ku quan shu* 續修四庫全書 in its full
length. In some pre-modern editions the author is given as Li Chunfeng 李淳
風. Yuan Tiangang 袁天罡 is said to have amended the text.

The text is divided into numerous *juan* 卷, each of them with a different title. For example, *juan* 1 has the title Qing xian qi fa 請仙箕法; *juan* 2: Liu jia tian

shu 六甲天書; *juan* 3: Bu tian ge jue 步天歌訣; and so on. As is characteristic of such folk manuscripts, the wording is often quite idiosyncratic.

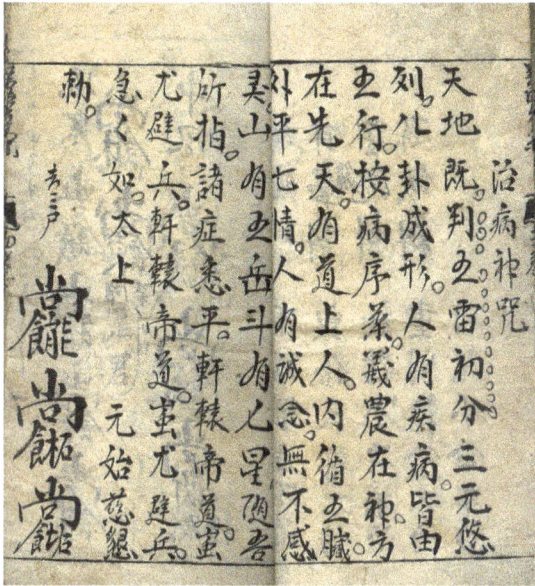

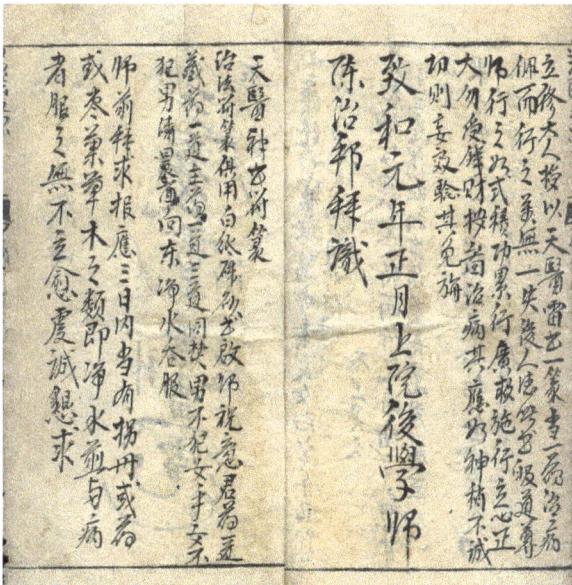

The present volume begins with a preface signed with a name "The master of physical genuineness, a man in the mountains with wet valleys", Han gu shan ren ti zhen zi 涵谷山人體真子. This is followed by an enumeration of

13 medical specialties, and a list of five conditions under which no treatment should take place. A subsequent long list of charms constructed from Chinese ordinary characters includes advice on pharmaceutical substances to be ingested together with the charms. The charms are mostly those with the character 尚 at their top. The drugs used to prepare a decoction for ingesting together with the charms follow the nature of the illness to be cured, and include 紫蘇、乳香、當歸、川芎、扁豆、茵陳、桃仁、薄荷、木香、陳皮, and 生薑.

The list of character-charms is followed by numerous pages with oral spells. Some of them are to be used for therapeutic purposes, others not. The oral spells are followed by 15 seal type charms, some of them with a comment specifying their therapeutic indications. They are followed by more than ten pages with character-style charms and, where applicable, their respective therapeutic indications, such as *shang feng ke sou* 傷風咳嗽, "harm caused by wind with cough", *she chong yao* 蛇蟲咬, "bites by snakes and bugs", and *xiao er ye ti* 小兒夜啼, "children crying during the night".

***

| | |
|---|---|
| TITLE: | (*Za chao* 雜抄, Copy of miscellaneous items) |
| ID: | 8907 |
| CONTENTS: | Pharmaceutical recipes |
| APPEARANCE: | A simple and crude manuscript volume of only a few pages, but above average calligraphy. No title |
| BINDING: | Originally paper spills. New cover with thread binding. |
| MEASURE: | 22.7 x 12.0 |
| TITLE PAGE: | No. No table of contents. |
| NO. OF PAGES: | 5 |
| L.P. /CH.L: | Very uneven |
| LAYOUT: | No lines, no frames |
| AUTHOR AND YEAR OF TEXT: | |
| | Unknown |
| YEAR OF COPY: | Republican era. |

SURVEY OF CONTENTS: Although this is a very simple manuscript volume, its contents are rather diverse. Paragraphs bearing the titles: Jia qu fan wu gui ri ge 嫁娶犯五鬼日歌, Sheng zi dui 生子對, Zu zong dui 祖宗對, Ban jia yue ge 搬家月歌, and An zao ri ge 安竈日歌 are not related to medical therapy. Other paragraphs offer advice on therapeutic issues, such as how to rescue "persons who have thrown themselves into a river or into a well", tou he tiao jing qiang jiu 投 河跳井, a folk prescription, *pian fang* 偏方, to treat injuries and bone fractures resulting from falls and blows, a *shui beng bing zheng hai fang* 水崩病症海方, another recipe for "injuries from falls and blows", *die da sun shang* 跌打損傷, a "recipe for lower back pain", *yao tong fang* 腰痛方, and a recipe for "a swollen neck, throat pain, and an inability to swallow", *zhong bo zi sang teng yan bu xia* 腫脖子嗓疼咽不下. The volume concludes with several recipes from regular Chinese medicine, in contrast to single ingredient folk recipes based on experience rather than theory.

***

TITLE:                 *Qi zhong bi you ke guan* 其中必有可觀, There must be some-
                       thing in it that should be looked at
ID:                    8908
CONTENTS:              Exorcism, pharmaceutical recipes
APPEARANCE:            Ancient manuscript volume. Edges and cover severely dam-
                       aged. Calligraphy above average. Cover inscription: 其中必
                       有可觀.
BINDING:               Thread
MEASURE:               19.5 x 12.9
TITLE PAGE:            No. No table of contents.
NO. OF PAGES:          32
L.P. /CH.L:            14 x approx. 27
LAYOUT:                No lines, no frames
AUTHOR AND YEAR OF TEXT:     Anonymous, Qing dynasty.
YEAR OF COPY:          Qing dynasty taboos on characters 玄 and 痰 strictly ob-
                       served. End of Qing dynasty.

SURVEY OF CONTENTS: This volume was written by an author with a relatively high level of formal education. The text has very few writing errors. The contents include both apotropaic and pharmaceutical approaches. The volume
begins with three patterns for oral incantations to be said by believers who
wish to establish a contact with the gods, in this case "Heavenly teacher Zhang
from Dragon and Tiger mountain in Jiangxi", jiang xi long hu shan zhang tian
shi 江西龍虎山張天師. The issues raised are losses in financial affairs. They are
followed by several examples of graphic charms, such as *feng tong fu* 封筒符,
"charm to close a pipe", and further sections with the titles: 天光法咒, 請神, 送
神, 使土地小鬼, 護身咒, and 五雷咒, as well as 圓光諜文, 飛行法, 緊箍咒法,
避兵, 避箭, 隱身, 鎮鬼, and 遣神. Most of these are accompanied by charm
drawings.

Only the following contents are more or less related to therapy. These are
recipes to treat choking, loss of consciousness and "heart qi pain", *xin qi tong* 心
氣痛. This includes rarely seen techniques such as *luo han xia ma sha* 羅漢下
馬沙, "Powder to make an arhat dismount from a horse", and *zhui hun pao* 追魂
炮, "cannon to chase the *hun* soul". These are not designed to cure diseases but
to protect one's body and ward off enemies. The ingredients to prepare the *luo
han xia ma sha* 羅漢下馬沙 are *sheng bi bo* 生蓽撥, *sheng chuan wu* 生川烏,

*sheng cao wu* 生草烏, *ba dou* 巴豆, *tong you* 桐油, and *mian sha* 麵沙. "All the pharmaceutical drugs are to be ground to a powder. This is to be evenly mixed with the *tong* oil. Then the flour is added. This is then to be dried in the sun until 80% dry. When it is to be applied, it is to be dispersed with the wind. When it hits [the victim], his eyes will be blinded. This can be reversed by rinsing with a decoction of *gan cao* 甘草." 先將諸藥為末，以桐油拌勻，再將麵

沙拌上，俟匀，日曬八分乾，用時在上風頭撒之，中則目瞎不見。解以甘草煎水洗. The ingredients for the *zhui hun pao* 追魂炮 include *chuan wu* 川烏, *cao wu* 草烏, *nao yang hua* 鬧楊花, *hu qie hua* 胡茄花, *xiong lang fen* 雄狼糞, and *ban mao* 斑蝥, 3 *qian* 錢 each. "These ingredients are powdered, then one adds 4 *liang* 兩 *liu huang* 硫黃, and prepares firecrackers. When a robber enters the house, they are ignited and thrown onto him. One must hold water in his own mouth to prevent oneself from being affected. It will be of no use if thrown down from somewhere high. Persons struck by the fumes will fall unconscious and do not wake up again unless one forces cold water into their mouth and spouts it into their face." 將諸藥為末，加硫黃四兩，裝成爆竹。遇有盜賊入房，點著擲出，必須自己含水一口，以防自迷。若自高擲下則不用矣。中烟之人昏迷不醒，以涼水灌口，噴面即醒。

The "song to make a disease retreat", *tui bing ge* 退病歌, is followed by more than 190 recipes. For the most part these are unsophisticated single ingredient folk recipes. Most of them are pharmaceutical recipes, some are apotropaic techniques. Examples of the former are the following:

心口疼　*xin kou teng*

一個烏梅兩個棗，　*yi ge wu me liang ge zao*

七個杏仁一齊搗。　*Qi ge xing ren yi qi tao*

男用黃酒女用醋，　*nan yong huang jiu nü yong cu*

吃了不疼直到老，　*chi le bu tent zhi dao lao*

"Pain in the stomach pit:

One dark plum, two dates

Seven almonds, pound together

For males use yellow wine, for women vinegar

Once ingested there will be no more pain till old age."

The "recipe to treat pain in the heart", *zhi xin teng fang* 治心疼方:

七粒胡椒三個棗 *qi li hu jiao san ge zao*，

五個杏仁一處搗。　*Wu ge xing ren yi chu dao*

搏成七丸燒酒送 *tuan cheng qi wan shao jiu song*

九種心痛俱能好 *jiu zhong xin tong ju neng hao*

„Seven pepper kernels, three dates.

Five almonds, pound together.

Form into seven pills and ingest them with brandy.

The nine types of pain in the heart will all be healed."

A "recipe for abortion", *duo tai fang* 墮胎方:

一巴豆，二紅娘， *yi ba dou er hong niang*

班毛三個加射香。 *Ban mao san ge jia she xiang*

射香一月用一分， *she xiang yi yue yong yi fen*

熱水送下去， *re shui song xia qu*

母子兩分張 *mu zi liang fen zhang*

One bean *ba dou*, two items *hong niang*,

Three pieces *ban mao*, add *she xiang*.

*She xiang* per month (of pregnancy) use 1 *fen*.

Ingest with hot water, and it will be discharged.

Mother and child will be separated.

Among the apotropaic recipes are some of great age. For example, the recipe 跑走不出境：將本人髮纏紡花車子抽（軸），即走不出 was recorded in the Tang dynasty *Ben cao shi yi* 本草拾遺. A recipe for abortion was veiled by the designation hai di chu bao fang 海底出寶方, "to release a treasure from the bottom of the seas". Its details are as follows: 紅娘四個，班毛七個，生半夏錢半，花粉二錢，黑丑半分，甘遂二錢，牙皂一錢，蔥白一科，金頭蜈蚣二條，共末，水為丸，絹包送入陰戶，加原香每月一分，見血即墜，"*hong niang*, four; *ban mao*, three; unprocessed *ban xia*, one half *qian*; *hua fen*, two *qian*; *hei chou*, one half *fen*, *gan sui*, two *qian*; *ya zao*, one *qian*. *Cong bai*, 1 *ke*. Gold head *wu song*, two. Powderize together. Use water to form pills. Wrap in gauze and insert into the yin gate. Add *yuan xiang*, 1 *fen* for each month [of pregnancy]. When blood appears [the fetus] will come down."

\*\*\*

| | |
|---|---|
| TITLE: | *Zhang Tianshi fu ji* 張天師符集, Collection of Celestial Master Zhang's charms |
| ID: | 8909 |
| CONTENTS: | Charms and spells |
| APPEARANCE: | Ancient manuscript volume. Initial pages lost. Paper darkened by age. Cover added by later hand. Inscription: 張天師符集. Average calligraphy. |
| BINDING: | Thread, later repaired with adhesive tape. |
| MEASURE: | 18.3 x 12.7 |
| TITLE PAGE: | No |

NO. OF PAGES:        40

L.P. /CH.L:          Pages without charms: Approx. 10 x 22

LAYOUT:              No lines, no frames

AUTHOR AND YEAR OF TEXT:

                     Unknown

YEAR OF COPY:        Character 玄 not written to observe a Qing dynasty taboo.

                     Republican era.

SURVEY OF CONTENTS: This is a collection of charms and oral spells. The contents are not directly related to the title "Collected charms of the Heavenly Teacher Zhang". Each charm is accompanied by an oral incantation. The titles of the charms are: 淨壇符、撮光符、光不圓符、定光符、請土地符、請灶君符、催神符、安神符、追魂符、定魂符、現像符、轉面符、驅魂符、送神符.

In addition, this volume includes ancient black magic, such as a "Minor technique to press down thieves and robbers", *zei dao xiao zhen shu* 賊盜小鎮術, and "Cut a physical appearance and use it to press down [somebody]", *jian xing yong zhen* 剪形用鎮. To apply these techniques a wooden human effigy is prepared which is then pierced with a needle. Or a person's name and birth date are written with cinnabar ink on the effigy's chest, and the effigy is then buried in a ditch. Such techniques were widespread among the people from Han times through the Qing dynasty.

In the middle of the volume a list of 90 finger gestures provides their designations and also, for most of them, advice on how to bend, stretch, and touch the fingers of both hands. The use of such gestures is not explained.

In its final section another 140 or more ideogram-type charms are drawn. Some of them have the same designation but look rather different. Some are accompanied by oral spells, others not.

***

| | |
|---|---|
| TITLE: | *Zhu you shi san ke* 祝由十三科, Specialty 13: Invocation of the origins. |
| ID: | 8910 |
| CONTENTS: | Exorcism |
| APPEARANCE: | Ancient manuscript volume. Cover made from tough paper; greyed over time. Inscription: 祝由十三科/壹本/癸卯年春□□/王記. Calligraphy above average. The text is written in a framework of vertical and horizontal lines drawn by pencil. |
| BINDING: | Thread |
| MEASURE: | 18.0 x 12.1 |
| TITLE PAGE: | No |
| NO. OF PAGES: | 23 |
| L.P. /CH.L: | 11 x approx. 21 |
| LAYOUT: | Upper and lower margins empty. Text written within a framework of horizontal lines above and below, and vertical lines between all columns of Chinese characters. |

AUTHOR AND YEAR OF TEXT:
                       Unknown

YEAR OF COPY:    Character 玄 not written to observe a Qing dynasty taboo.
                       Republican era.

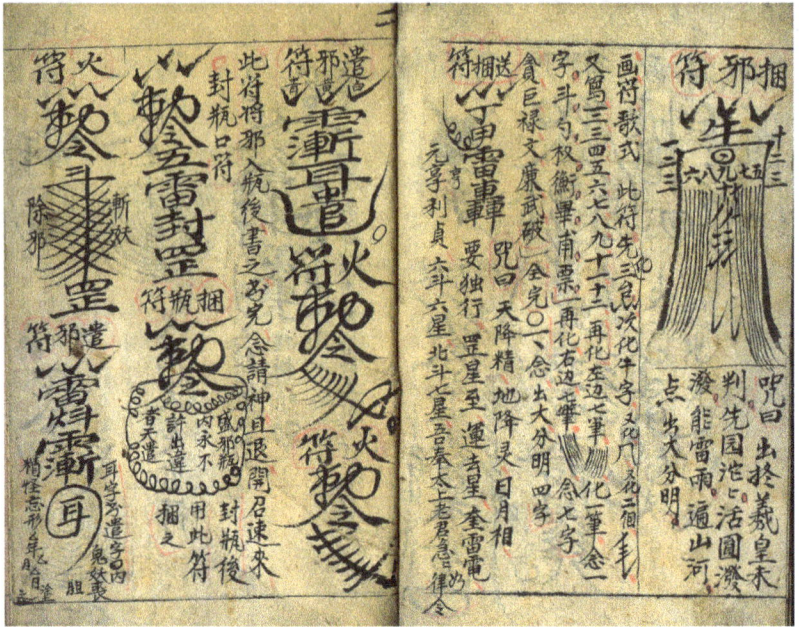

SURVEY OF CONTENTS: Title and contents do not agree. A title like "Incantation of the origins, the 13th specialty", *Zhu you shi san ke* 祝由十三科, should be devoted to apotropaic therapy of illness. This is not the case. The charms recorded in this volume serve diverse purposes pursued by Daoist masters.

The text begins with a "Pattern to ask for a meeting", *yao hui fa* 邀會法, which is designed "to call upon a fox spirit", *qing hu xian* 請狐仙. Allegedly, this technique enables one to attract a beautiful fox spirit which will then follow the requests of the magician, including marrying him. To achieve this end various incantations and charms are to be applied, such as "to invite a fox", *qing hu* 請狐, "to have a fox descend", *jiang hu* 降狐, "to lock up a fox", *suo hu* 鎖狐, "to open the lock", *jie suo* 解鎖, and "to send off the fox", *song hu* 送狐.

Next is a section Fu yao suo xie shen jing guai 縛妖鎖邪神精怪, "to tie up demons and to lock up evil spirits and demonic essence", with 17 charms for use against: *ji jing* 雞精, "chicken essence/spirit"; *she jing* 蛇精, "snake essence/spirit"; *hu li jing* 狐狸精, "fox essence/spirit"; *mao jing* 貓精, "cat essence/spirit"; *shu jing* 樹精, "tree essence/spirit"; *ha ma jing* 蛤蟆精, "frog essence/spirit"; *hou jing* 猴精; "monkey essence/spirit"; *zhu jing* 豬精, "hog essence/spirit"; *hua jing* 花精, "flower essence/spirit"; *gou jing* 狗精, "dog essence/spirit"; *huang jing* 黃 精, "yellow essence/spirit"; *xie zi jing* 蝎子精, "scorpion essence/spirit"; *shu jing* 鼠精, "mouse essence/spirit"; *shi jing* 石精, "stone essence/spirit"; *gui jing* 鬼精, "demon essence/spirit". There is also a *zhuan zhuo zi fa* 轉桌子法, "a technique to make a table rotate".

Some of the techniques recorded in this volume serve to cause trouble of one kind or another. An example is the "method for steaming buns", *zheng sheng bo bo fa* 蒸生餑餑法. Allegedly it can be used to thwart a person's attempt to prepare steamed buns in a steamer. Other paragraphs bear titles such as *duan jue shu fa* 斷絕鼠法, "method to sever mice"; *yan jing zhou* 壓精咒, "method to press down essence/spirits"; *jiu long hua gu fa* 九龍化骨法, "nine tiger meth-od to transform bones"; *ri xing qian li bu juan fa* 日行千里不倦法, "method to daily march a thousand miles without being tired", and *tao fu zhuo zei fa* 桃符 捉賊法, "method to capture robbers with a peach wood charm". These sections have no therapeutic purposes, in contrast to a few other sections such as *cui shen fu shi* 催生符式, "amulets to hasten delivery"; *zhi nüe ji fu* 治瘧疾符, "am-ulets to cure malaria illness"; *zhi ya teng zhou* 治牙疼咒, "incantation to treat toothache".

The final part of the volume lists commonly used charms, named 請神符、 圓光法、土地符、五雷符、護身符、捉鬼符、降邪符、斬邪符、貶邪符、 捆邪符、遣邪符、除邪符、鎖邪符、治鬼符、雷符、翻天、覆地.

***

| | |
|---|---|
| TITLE: | *Yuan guang ji yao* 圓光集要, A collection of essentials from the radiance emanating from the head |
| ID: | 8911 |
| CONTENTS: | Charms and spells |
| APPEARANCE: | Simple ancient manuscript volume. Cover missing. A torn blank title page left. No title inscription. Text complete. Heading of first section Yuan guang ji yao 圓光集要 used here as title of the entire volume. Writing in minute charac-ters. Good calligraphy. |
| BINDING: | Paper spills |
| MEASURE: | 19.7 x 13.0 |
| TITLE PAGE: | Blank |

NO. OF PAGES:     27

L.P. /CH.L:     Approx. 14 x 25

LAYOUT:     No lines, no frames

AUTHOR AND YEAR OF TEXT:

    Anonymous, Qing dynasty.

YEAR OF COPY:   End of Qing dynasty. The character 玄 is always written with
                the final stroke omitted. Also, the text includes references to
                the *guang xu* 光緒 reign period.

SURVEY OF CONTENTS: This is a Daoist's collection of charms. Their designations are: 淨壇符式、撮光符、催光符、光亮符、定光符、請神符、催神
符、安神符、追魂符、驅魂符、拘灶君、五雷符. They widely exceed the
realm of therapeutics, and may be used for all kinds of activities performed by
Daoist practitioners. The present volume is special in that it documents several
magic techniques to be used for arranging a marriage, such as the *lian yin fu
shi* 連姻符式, "amulets for linking a marriage"; *he mei fu shi* 合美符式, "amulets for a union with a beauty"; *kun he fu shi* 坤合符式, "amulets for bringing
a female into a union". Other techniques bear titles such as *jie yuan* 解冤, "to
clear wrongs"; *duan qiao* 斷橋, "to break a bridge" (advice on how to kill a river
demon by forming his paper effigy, place it on a paper bridge, and burn it) ; *qu
yi* 驅縊, "to expel [the demon of someone who was forced to commit suicide
by] hanging"; *shui gui* 水鬼, "[to destroy a] water demon", and *du sheng* 毒害,
"[to save someone from] poisoning [by inappropriate medication]". They serve
to cope with injustice and death by accident. A technique *jiang xie guang* 降
邪光 is supposed to assist in cases of accidents brought about by demons. The
number of spells devoted to therapy is very small. Examples are *zhi bing fu shi*
治病符式, *yuan yin fu* 元引符, and *ji bing fu* 疾病符.

   Seen in comparison with other such volumes, although the present volume
is rather thin it nevertheless includes some unique contents.

***

TITLE:          *Tian shi shen fu zhi bai bing zhen bai shi xiong* 天師神符治百
                病鎮百事兇, Divine charms of the heavenly teachers to cure
                a hundred diseases, and to suppress all types of atrocities.
ID:             8912
CONTENTS:       Charms and spells
APPEARANCE:     Simple ancient manuscript volume. Cover made from cot-
                ton paper. Inscription: 天師神符治百病鎮百事兇/龐寇記.
                Calligraphy below average. Large characters.
BINDING:        Paper spills
MEASURE:        20.0 x 11.0

TITLE PAGE:        No. No table of contents.
NO. OF PAGES:      11
L.P. /CH.L:        Uneven. Mostly 3 columns of charms. <15 ch. /line.
LAYOUT:            Each page with frame 17.2 x 9.0. Horizontal and vertical
                   lines drawn by hand.
AUTHOR AND YEAR OF TEXT:
                   Unknown
YEAR OF COPY:      Paper quality suggests Republican era.

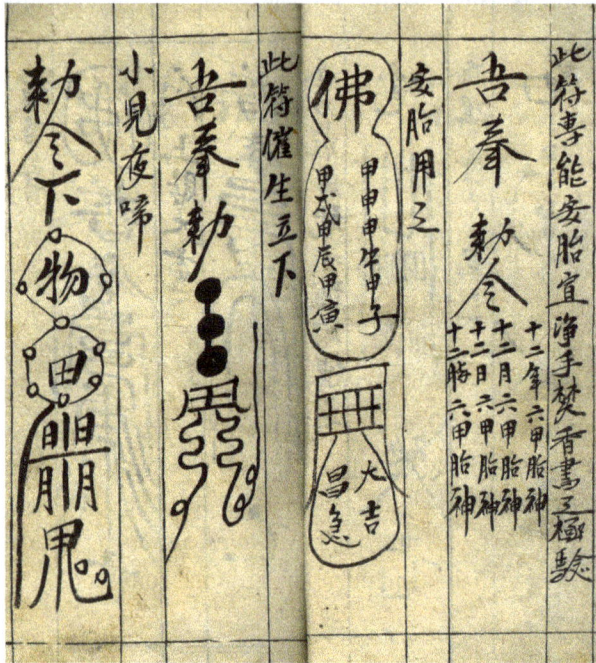

SURVEY OF CONTENTS: This is a record of 56 charms with mostly very brief and simple annotations concerning therapeutic and other indications, but without oral spells. Each charm is accompanied by only one sentence, giving its name and explaining its therapeutic function. Some of these indications are rather broad, e.g., *chu xie bao ming* 除邪保命, "drive away evil and rescue a life", 鎮宅, 邪不敢侵, 、小鬼一切神煞、邪魔鬼怪、治百事、大吉、分家不利、財物不旺、六畜損傷、治百病. Others are very specifically designed to cure a particular ailment, such as 頭疼、風頭、火眼、瘡瘤、安胎、催生、小兒夜啼、腹痛、心驚、睡臥不安. The range of issues dealt with is rather limited. Apparently, the person who wrote this manuscript volume did not enjoy a high level of formal education.

\*\*\*

| | |
|---|---|
| TITLE: | *Kai yan jing* 開眼經, Classic to open the eyes |
| ID: | 8913 |
| CONTENTS: | Education reading primer |
| APPEARANCE: | Simple, poor, ancient manuscript volume. Thin paper mulberry paper cover. Inscription: 開眼經/王重鈞. Several characters scribbled for exercise, without specific meaning: 丁卯、己卯、十八、經. Inside front cover inscription 開眼經 repeated. |
| BINDING: | Originally paper spills. Thread binding added by later hand. |
| MEASURE: | 19.4 x 11.7 |
| TITLE PAGE: | Inside front cover, inscription 开眼經 |
| NO. OF PAGES: | 27 |
| L.P. /CH.L: | 6 x 16 |
| LAYOUT: | No lines, no frames |
| AUTHOR AND YEAR OF TEXT: | |
| | Wei Tang 唯堂, 1710. Copyist: Wang Zhongjun 王重鈞. |
| YEAR OF COPY: | Character 玄 written to observe a Qing dynasty taboo. End of Qing dynasty. |

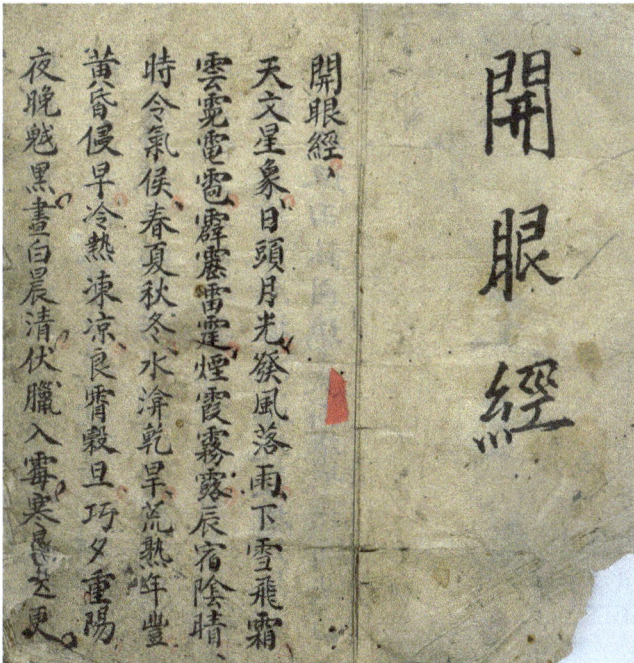

SURVEY OF CONTENTS: The *Kai yan jing* 開眼經 is an ancient primer used in the education of young boys. The meaning of *kai yan* 開眼, lit. "to open the eyes", and *qi meng* 啓蒙, "to arise from a dream/ignorance" is identical. Both are used for the earliest formal education of boys. The present volume does not have an author's name and a date. According to the internet, a wan juan lou cang 萬卷樓藏 has published a *Kai yan jing* 開眼經. The preface states: 康熙庚寅歲蒲月上澣唯堂父編次. The year *kang xi, geng yin* 康熙庚寅 is the 49th year of the *kang xi* reign period, i.e., 1710. Another edition was issued in Anhui 安徽 by 屯溪菇古堂書坊.

The present volume resembles the *Qian zi wen* 千字文; it is rhymed with four character lines. It begins with *tian wen xing xiang* 天文星象, *ri tou yue guang* 日頭月光 ... and ends with *nong zhang nong wa* 弄璋弄瓦, *bao ge kann sheng* 報個看生, covering more than 5.100 characters. The themes covered include: natural climate, geological environment, family and generations, social structure, professions and nationalities, the body and its parts, architecture and traffic infrastructure, items used in daily life, all types of tools, cooking utensils and farm tools, things associated with agriculture, grains and vegetables, fruit and victuals, land and sea animals, illnesses and pharmaceutical drugs, etc. Only the section "illnesses and pharmaceutical drugs", *ji bing yao wu* 疾病藥物, is related to medical therapy. This section has 410 characters and introduces more than 60 disease names and 136 pharmaceutical substances. The text of this section constitutes one twelfth of the entire text, showing the degree of signifance associated with this vocabulary.

***

| | |
|---|---|
| TITLE: | *Jing yan liang fang* 經驗良方, Proven, good recipes |
| ID: | 8914 |
| CONTENTS: | Pharmaceutical recipes |
| APPEARANCE: | Ancient manuscript volume. Kraft paper cover with oil stains. Inscription upper left: 經驗良方. Inscription on bottom edge: 光緒卅年夏. Average calligraphy. |
| BINDING: | Thread |
| MEASURE: | 22.0 x 15.2 |
| TITLE PAGE: | No |
| NO. OF PAGES: | 77 |
| L.P. /CH.L: | 10 x approx. 23 |

LAYOUT: Red dividing lines washed out by air humidity and no longer clearly marked.

AUTHOR AND YEAR OF TEXT: Anonymous, Qing dynasty

YEAR OF COPY: 1904

SURVEY OF CONTENTS: This is a list of more than 460 pharmaceutical recipes, ordered along different illnesses. These clusters are indicated with small script at the outer margins for easy thumbing through the volume. Initially, prior to therapeutic indications the text provides data on vessel movement, on disease dynamics, on therapeutic patterns and the application of a recipe. Further in the volume these informations diminish and become very simple. Disease dynamics and pathological conditions are no longer explained in detail. The illness groups covered are the following: 翻胃、氣瘰、小便、大便、吐血、衄血、咳嗽痰血、嘔血、婦人逆行經、咳嗽、氣鼓、遺精、淋瀝、婦人陰挺、婦女干血、男子白濁、精滑不禁、偏墜、腎囊風、陰戶病症下寒、小兒赤游丹、白癜風、痰迷不醒、拔牙、長乳斷經、小兒痞塊、眼科、牙疳、百病丸藥、小便出屎、痢疾、小兒痢疾口瘡肚脹目腫、室女大症、吹喉、內外痔、婦人積快、腰疼、腿疼、心疼、肚疼、小腸疝氣、治蟲ㄚ、追風膏、婦人陰瘡、頭疼、雜症專治方 (the recommendation of "black gold powder", *wu jin san* 烏金散, for treating "bird's nest sores", *yan wo chuang* 燕窩瘡, is illustrated by a drawing of the latter.). In the final section recipes are listed without reference to the name of an illness. Apparently, they were recorded as they came to the attention of the volume's author. A small number of recipes are single ingredient formulae. Some are to be used for abortion, others as contraceptiva for long-lasting sterilization, and there are a few from the realm of veterinary medicine.

***

| | |
|---|---|
| TITLE: | (*Jia yong yao fang* 家用藥方, Pharmaceutical recipes for home use) |
| ID: | 8915 |
| CONTENTS: | Pharmaceutical recipes |
| APPEARANCE: | Ancient manuscript volume. Locally produced tissue paper. Cover destroyed. Handwriting by numerous persons but one person responsible for much of the contents. His calligraphy is very specific and beautiful. |
| BINDING: | Thread |
| MEASURE: | 19.9 x 19.7 |
| TITLE PAGE: | No |
| NO. OF PAGES: | 47 |
| L.P. /CH.L: | 10-12 x 10-13 |

LAYOUT:              No lines, no frames
AUTHOR AND YEAR OF TEXT:
                     Anonymous, recent.
YEAR OF COPY:   Character 玄 not written to observe a Qing dynasty taboo.
                Republican era.

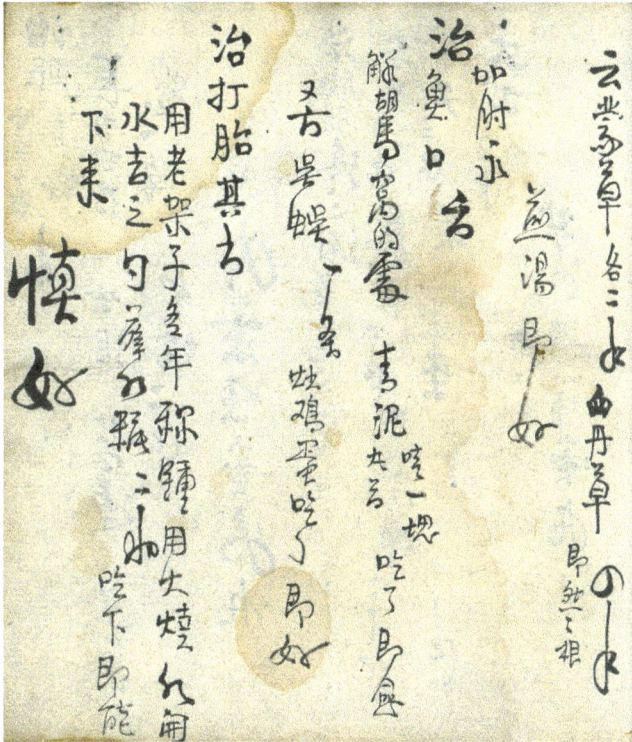

SURVEY OF CONTENTS: This volume is a list of pharmaceutical recipes as they
are transmitted among the common people. Often the person from whom a
recipe was obtained is mentioned, for example, 二嫂說, "told by second elder
brother's wife", 老五說, "told by 5th brother", 買瓜客說, "told by client who pur-
chased a melon", 蒲城文廟前裕隆書局印, "printed by the *yu long* book store
in front of the literature temple in Pucheng", 窯上敬思他舅父開方與官印子
用、振西說此方, "this recipe was prescribed by Jingsi of Yaoshang for use by
officials, and it was told by Zhenxi". Still the initial part of this volume was
copied as a whole. The handwriting there is coherent. Apparently, this early
part was copied by one person from another person's private records. Later on,
the copyist himself continued to collect and record further recipes. Hence, this

volume may be seen as a model of how such personal folk recipe collections developed. In fact, this is a typical example of a folk record of recipes.

As the early part was copied from one source, it has a certain structure. At the beginning the author recorded several recipes from veterinary medicine, with some recipes for human therapy interspersed. Next are 107 recipes for women's ailments, including at least one recipe for abortion, then 120 recipes for various ailments and urgent cases, and at the end 75 recipes as casual notes, without therapeutic indication.

\*\*\*

| TITLE: | (*Wu jin san* 烏金散, Black gold powder) |
|---|---|
| ID: | 8916 |
| CONTENTS: | Gynecology |
| APPEARANCE: | Ancient manuscript volume. Cover damaged. No title. Excellent handwriting. Large, beautiful characters. |
| BINDING: | Paper spills |
| MEASURE: | 23.3 x 13.1 |
| TITLE PAGE: | No |
| NO. OF PAGES: | 21 |
| L.P. /CH.L: | No lines, no frames |
| LAYOUT: | 8 x 16 |
| AUTHOR AND YEAR OF TEXT: | |
| | Anonymous, late Qing dynasty. |
| YEAR OF COPY: | The character 玄 is not written with the final stroke omitted. Also, the paper is of more recent quality. Republican era. |

SURVEY OF CONTENTS: This volume is a record of pharmaceutical recipes. The largest section has the title Wu jin san zhi tai qian chan hou zhu bing 烏金散治胎前産後諸病, "The Black Gold Powder to cure all diseases during pregnancy and following delivery". The Black Gold Powder, *wu jin san* 烏金散, is prepared with the following constituents: *peng e zhu* 蓬莪朮, *shou di huang* 熟地黄, *chi shao yao* 赤芍藥, *xiong hei dou* 雄黑豆, *dang gui* 當歸, *gan jiang* 乾薑, *pu huang* 蒲黄, *hong hua* 紅花, *guan gui* 官桂. These nine substances are powderized and then ingested with different liquids in accordance with different therapeutic indications. Following this recipe are 18 discourses, *lun* 論, on the causes of all types of ailments encountered during pregnancy and following delivery. This includes advice on pharmaceutical substances to be added to (and boiled together with) or taken away from the original Black Gold Powder formula as required by different diseases. Finally, there is a rhymed statement on each of these diseases repeating the meaning behind the application of the drugs mentioned above.

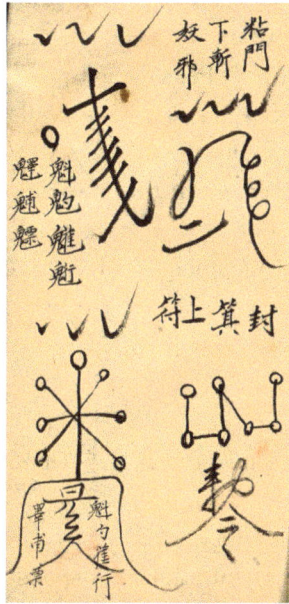

The Black Gold Powder is a cure-all formula introduced into Chinese traditional gynecology towards the end of the Qing dynasty. The same recipe was also applied as pills. The core recipe could be modified by adding or omitting substances in accordance with the individual pathological condition of a patient. During the Qing dynasty numerous books were published to elucidate the effects of Black Gold Powder. The current volume introduces the powder variation of Black Gold Powder; we have not found a printed original from which the present text may have been copied.

The section on the Black Gold Powder is preceded by two brief paragraphs on Celestial Stems and Five Phases, *tian gan wu xing* 天干五行, and Earth Branches and Five Phases, *di zhi wu xing* 地支五行, as well as 15 recipes for various ailments. Following the section on the Black Gold Powder, another two pharmaceutical recipes are documented, as well as 25 charms to ward off evil.

*\*\*\**

| | |
|---|---|
| TITLE: | *Yan ke liang fang* 眼科良方, Good recipes in ophthalmology |
| ID: | 8917 |
| CONTENTS: | Ophthalmology |
| APPEARANCE: | Ancient manuscript volume of good quality. Cover without title. Inscription: 凡借看者看畢即送原主是禱/溫氏置/晋峰子遠敬抄. Text written in beautiful characters; careful handwriting. |
| BINDING: | Paper spills |
| MEASURE: | 23.7 x 13.8 |
| TITLE PAGE: | No |
| NO. OF PAGES: | 18 |
| L.P. /CH.L: | No lines, no frames |
| LAYOUT: | 8 x 16 |
| AUTHOR AND YEAR OF TEXT: | |
| | Wen Jingfeng 溫晋峰, Ziyuan 子遠. Qing dynasty. |
| YEAR OF COPY: | An inscription towards the end of the volume reads: 同治九年冬月朔浣日晋峰子遠敬抄. Hence this volume was copied in 1870. |

SURVEY OF CONTENTS: This is a complete copy of the *Yan ke liang fang* 眼科良方, published in the 25th year of the *daoguang* 道光 reign period [1845]. The book is attributed to the Qing author Ye Tianshi 葉天士. The fact is, that it is a reprint of the Ming author Cheng Songya's 程松崖 *Yan ke jing yan liang fang* 眼科經驗良方 under Ye Tianshi's name. The text is extremely succinct. It begins with a drawing of an eye with segments identified as associated with the five long-term depots. This drawing is followed by an enumeration of 21 ailments of the eyes, each with a (mostly identical) drawing of an eye, a listing of the pathological conditions associated with this ailment, and an advice on which pharmaceutical recipe is to be used for treatment. At the end of the volume several recipes based on experience are recorded, and a recipe allegedly given, in the reign period *yuan feng* 元豐 of the Song dynasty, to a Prefect, *tai shou* 太守, for rinsing his eyes. This book was widely distributed and often copied by the people.

\*\*\*

| | |
|---|---|
| TITLE: | (*Jiu chao yao fang* 舊抄藥方; Ancient copy of pharmaceutical recipes) |
| ID: | 8918 |
| CONTENTS: | Pharmaceutical recipes |
| APPEARANCE: | Simple, ancient manuscript volume. Edges rubbed. Cover stained and at the lower bottom with a seal that is illegible. Inferior calligraphy. No title. |
| BINDING: | Paper spills |
| MEASURE: | 21.5 x 14.4 |
| TITLE PAGE: | No |
| NO. OF PAGES: | 19 |
| L.P. /CH.L: | 8 x 15-18 |
| LAYOUT: | No lines, no frames |
| AUTHOR AND YEAR OF TEXT: | |
| | Unknown |
| YEAR OF COPY: | The character 弦 is written with the final stroke omitted. The character 痰 is written with the lower 火 changed to 又. Late Qing dynasty. |

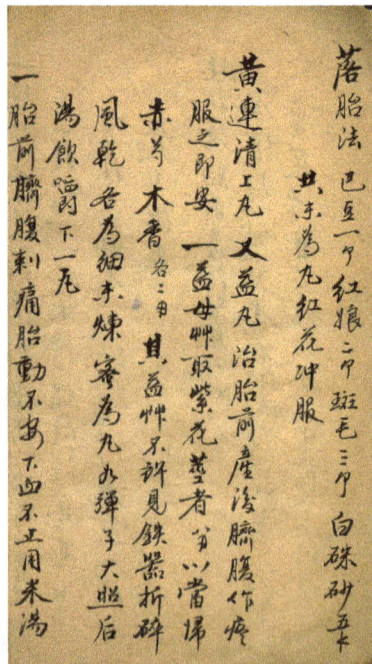

SURVEY OF CONTENTS: This is a record of 75 pharmaceutical recipes, including one apotropaic recipe, and one recipe from veterinary medicine. Most of the recipes are for ailments of women listed following no recognizable order. There are also recipes for strengthening male sexual potency (*jin qiang bu dao* 金槍不倒, "the golden rifle does not tip"; *xing yang fang* 醒陽方, "recipe to awaken the yang"), and recipes for abortion: *zhi wu liu ge tai bai fa bai zhong* 治五六個胎百發百中, "To treat five, six fetuses. One hundred usages, one hundred hits", with ingredients *ban mao* 斑毛, *hong niang* 紅娘, *ba dou shuang* 巴豆霜, *qing fen* 輕粉, *bai zhu sha* 白硃砂, *sheng she* 生射 (麝), and *zhu sha* 硃砂, and *luo tai fang* 落胎方, "recipe to drop the fetus", with *ba dou* 巴豆, *hong niang* 紅娘, *ban mao* 斑毛, and *bai zhu sha* 白硃砂. The number of recipes recorded is limited, and the writing was by several hands. Towards the end of the volume the handwriting is increasingly careless and deficient.

*** 

| | |
|---|---|
| TITLE: | *Ying zhou shi yong za ben* 應酬使用雜本, Volume on various issues associated with social intercourse |
| ID: | 8919 |
| CONTENTS: | Miscellaneous household needs |

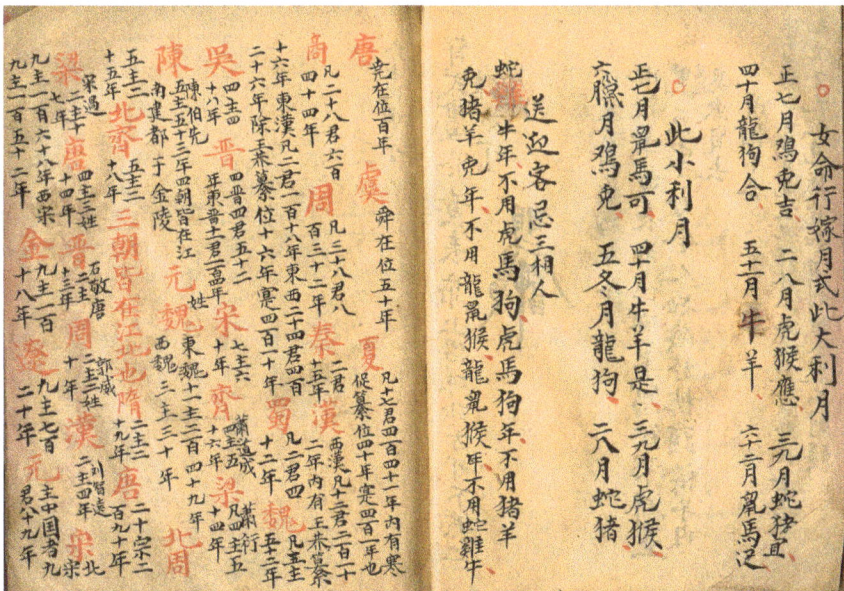

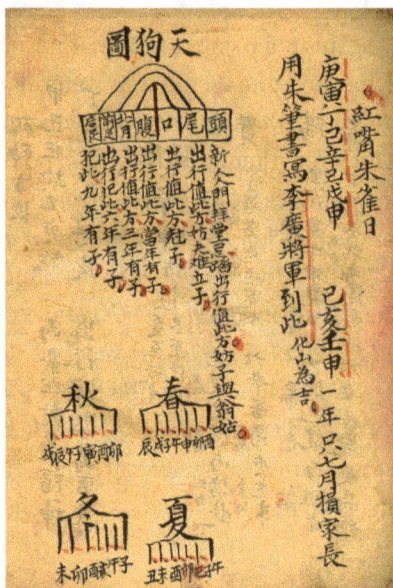

APPEARANCE:     Ancient manuscript volume. Cover stained and damaged. Lower left edge missing. Average calligraphy. Upper left inscription: 應酬使用雜本卷. To the right, inscription: 此本有老鼠方/楊學曾記. A recipe for rat ulcers is recorded on the back cover.

BINDING:        Thread

MEASURE:        16.3 x 12.8

TITLE PAGE:     Yes, with inscription: 應酬使用雜本小不求人/光緒貳拾伍年巧月貳拾貳日立/己亥年製/楊學曾記.

NO. OF PAGES:   29

L.P. /CH.L:     10-12 x 15-18

LAYOUT:         No lines, no frames

AUTHOR AND YEAR OF TEXT:

                Yang Xuehui 楊學曾, late Qing.

YEAR OF COPY:   Successively written from the 25th year of the *guang xu* 光緒 reign period, 1899, through the early years of the Republican era.

SURVEY OF CONTENTS: The title of this volume indicates that it is not concerned with medical-pharmaceutical contents in the first place. The first 14 pages have patterns to be used when writing letters or documents related to a wedding, 婚單、回親、請媒、請帖、媒人帖、慶壽帖、祭帖、還願、賣

地、立招字式、求雨表文. After these 14 pages the contents are quite diverse. They include charms (for treating an inadvertent ingestion of needles, or fish bones, bites by rabies dog, stings by scorpions, and for reducing pests such as rats and bedbugs), a list of dynasties, the 60 celestial stems and earth branches, a table of the mutual generation and destruction of the Five Phases, the eight trigrams, the 12 animals of the Zodiac, etc. All these tables and data are to be used for prognosis of lucky dates guiding one's life. Of immediate use for treatment there is only the "recipe to cure rat ulcers", *zhi lao shu chuang fang* 治老 鼠瘡方, recorded on the back of the title page.

*** 

| TITLE: | (*Za fang* 雜方, miscellaneous recipes) |
| --- | --- |
| ID: | 8920 |
| CONTENTS: | Pharmaceutical recipes |
| APPEARANCE: | Simple ancient manuscript volume. No front cover. Calligraphy deficient. Handwriting careless. |
| BINDING: | Paper spills |
| MEASURE: | 20.6 x 12.7 |
| TITLE PAGE: | No |
| NO. OF PAGES: | 17 |
| L.P. /CH.L: | 5-7 x 21 |

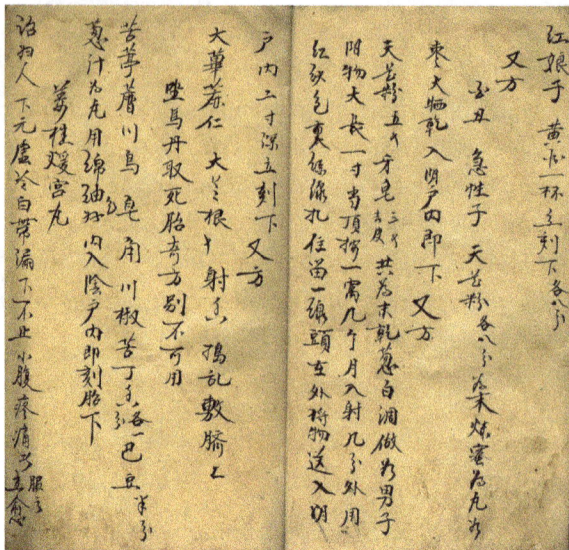

LAYOUT: No lines, no frames

AUTHOR AND YEAR OF TEXT: Unknown

YEAR OF COPY: The quality of the paper suggests that this volume dates from the Republican era.

SURVEY OF CONTENTS: This volume is a record of 36 pharmaceutical recipes. It includes more than ten recipes that would not be found in printed literature. At the very beginning several recipes for abortion are documented: 打胎方、下胎散、破血打胎湯、絕孕方、打胎方、又方、又方、又方, and also a recipe to deliver a dead fetus: 坐馬丹取死胎奇方. Such a large number of recipes for abortion, all listed together, is rarely seen. One example is as follows:

天花粉五錢，牙皂三個去皮，共為末，乾蔥白調做如男子陽物大，長一寸，當頂按一窩，幾個月入射（麝）幾分，外用紅紗包裹，絲線扎住，留一線在外，將物送入陰戶內二寸深，立刻下。

"Five *qian* of *tian hua fen* and three pieces of *ya zao*, with skin removed, are to be powderized together. Form a dried onion into the shape of the male member, with a length of 1 inch. At the tip press a dent into it which is to be filled with as many *fen* of musk as months for which the pregnancy has already lasted. Cover this with red gauze and fix this with silk threads. One thread should remain free. Then this is to be inserted into the vagina, two inches deep. [The fetus] will come down immediately."

There is also a recipe to "make a beautiful person drop her cloths", *mei ren tuo yi* 美人脱衣, to be used as a sexual stimulant. Another recipe advises on the application of a *meng yao* 蒙藥, lit. "Mongol drug", an abbreviation of the more commonly used term *meng han yao* 蒙汗藥, "Mongol sweat drug". This is, in fact, a knock-out narcotic used by robbers to drug their victims. The recipe is as follows:

"*tian ling gai* 天靈蓋, *nao yang hua* 鬧陽花, *bai zhi* 白芷, *cang zhu* 蒼朮, *tai bao* 胎包, *hai long* 海龍, *hai ma* 海馬, *shu fen* 鼠糞, *ji ju zi* 雞巨子, *shu wei* 鼠尾, *zi ding xiang* 紫丁香, *cun xiang* 寸香, *pu huang* 蒲黃, *sha mu tan* 杉木炭, *liu huang* 硫黃, *gong ji guan* 公雞管各, each 3 *qian*, prepare a fine powder and apply. To be used externally."

\*\*\*

| | |
|---|---|
| TITLE: | *Huo sheng pian* 護生篇, An essay on how to preserve life |
| ID: | 8921 |
| CONTENTS: | Gynecology |
| APPEARANCE: | Ancient manuscript volume. Average calligraphy. Cover with inscription: 護生篇/同治八年十一月十七日立/紀. |
| BINDING: | Thread |
| MEASURE: | 21.8 x 13.8 |
| TITLE PAGE: | No |
| NO. OF PAGES: | 21 |
| L.P. /CH.L: | 9 x approx. 20 |
| LAYOUT: | No lines, no frames |
| AUTHOR AND YEAR OF TEXT: | |
| | Qing, ca. 1798; Li Changke 李長科. |
| YEAR OF COPY: | The writer failed to observe the Qing taboo on the character 玄 and did not omit the final stroke. However, in folk manuscripts these imperial taboos were not always strictly observed. The present manuscript was written in the 8th year of the *tong zhi* 同治 reign period, i.e., in 1869. |

SURVEY OF CONTENTS: This volume focuses on women's ailments during pregnancy and following delivery. The title *Huo sheng pian* 護生篇 suggests that it may have been copied from a book of this title first published by the Qing author Li Changke 李長科 during the *dao guang* 道光 reign period under the title *Tai chan huo sheng pian* 胎產護生篇. The present volume begins with a recipe "elixir to snatch life as transmitted by the immortals", *xian chuan tuo ming dan* 仙傳奪命丹. This is followed by miscellaneous pharmaceutical recipes for therapeutic indications such as 產後血暈、達生、保胎、安胎、束胎、救生、難產、產後多種疾病、新生兒救護. Altogether these are 70 recipes.

*** 

| | |
|---|---|
| TITLE: | *Nan nü jing yan liang fang fu lu yan ke* 男女經驗良方附錄眼科, Proven, good recipes for males and females, with an appendix on ophthalmology |
| ID: | 8922 |
| CONTENTS: | Pharmaceutical recipes; ophthalmology |
| APPEARANCE: | Ancient manuscript volume. Cover severely damaged. Edges with some tear and wear. Cover inscription: 男女經驗良方附錄眼科/馬光裕堂置. Two personal seals with partly readable characters: 馬永祚印 and [ ]州圖印. Average calligraphy. Pages show many later comments inserted into the margins above, to the side and below the main text. |
| BINDING: | Thread |
| MEASURE: | 21.7 x 13.5 |
| TITLE PAGE: | No |
| NO. OF PAGES: | 39 |
| L.P. /CH.L: | 9 x 24 |
| LAYOUT: | No lines, no frames |
| AUTHOR AND YEAR OF TEXT: | Unknown |
| YEAR OF COPY: | The back of the front cover has some phonetic notations, suggesting that this volume is not very old. An inscription on the first page reads: 丙寅九月十五日起抄，廿一日止，七日成功. Hence this volumes dates from 1926. It was prepared by Ma Yongzuo 馬永祚. |

SURVEY OF CONTENTS: The contents of this volume consist of two parts. The main part consists of 131 pharmaceutical recipes, including one apotropaic formula. Most of these recipes, including typical recipes for abortion, are folk recipes commonly used by the people. Also, most are directed at illnesses; only very few are fixed recipes designed to tonify a person.

The second part is on ophthalmology. It begins with a preface identified as Guang xu wu yin Sun Muxian xu 光緒戊寅孫沐賢敘, "Narrative by Sun Muxian in the year *wu yin* of the *guang xu* reign period". Here one learns that this part is a copy of the *Ye Tianshi yan ke fang* 葉天士眼科方, published under the name of Ye Tianshi 葉天士. This is in fact Su Muxian's 孫沐賢 *Liang fang yan ke he bian* 良方眼科合編, which was then published as *Ye Tianshi yan ke fang* 葉天士眼科方. Another edition of this work was illegitimately published under the title *Cheng Songya xian sheng yan ke* 程松崖先生眼科. The special feature of this text is a listing of ten different ailments of the eyes, each case illustrated by a drawing of an eye with differing pathological features. For each condition an explanation is given, and pharmaceutical drugs are recommended for treatment. This book was frequently copied during the Qing dynasty and achieved a wide-spread distribution.

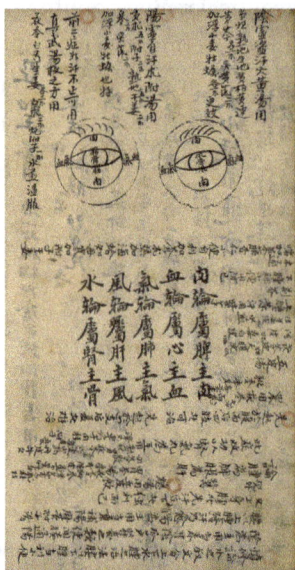

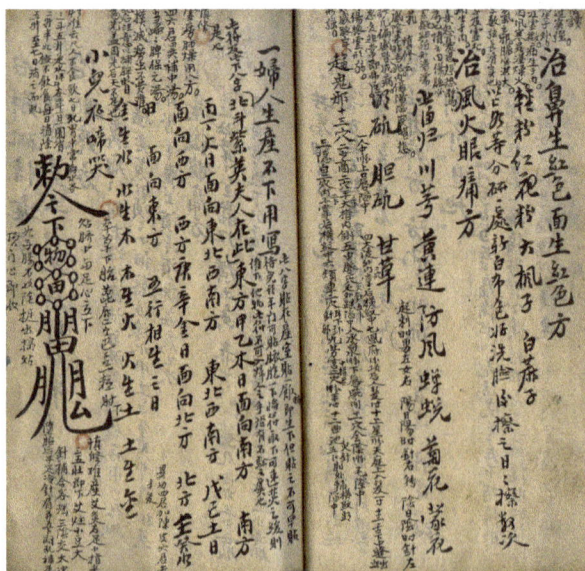

\*\*\*

| | |
|---|---|
| TITLE: | *Die da sun shang* 跌打損傷, Injuries from falls and blows. |
| ID: | 8923 |
| CONTENTS: | Traumatology |
| APPEARANCE: | Ancient manuscript volume with dark blue cloth cover thread bound around original paper cover. Front with two paper labels pasted on the cloth cover. Inscriptions: 跌打損傷 and 乾隆伍年. The text written on paper made from bamboo. Average calligraphy. Front of original paper cover with inscription: 祖傳秘方/跌打損傷. |
| BINDING: | Thread |
| MEASURE: | 19.2 x 13.5 |
| TITLE PAGE: | No |
| NO. OF PAGES: | 71 |
| L.P. /CH.L: | 8 x 14 |
| LAYOUT: | No lines, no frames |
| AUTHOR AND YEAR OF TEXT: | |
| | Unknown, Qing dynasty. |
| YEAR OF COPY: | The quality of the paper, the ink, and the non-observance of taboos suggest that this volume was written in the Republican era. |

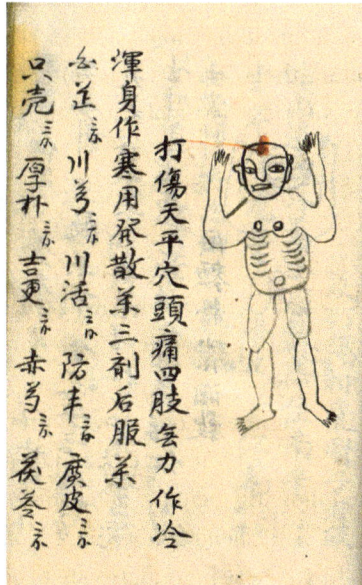

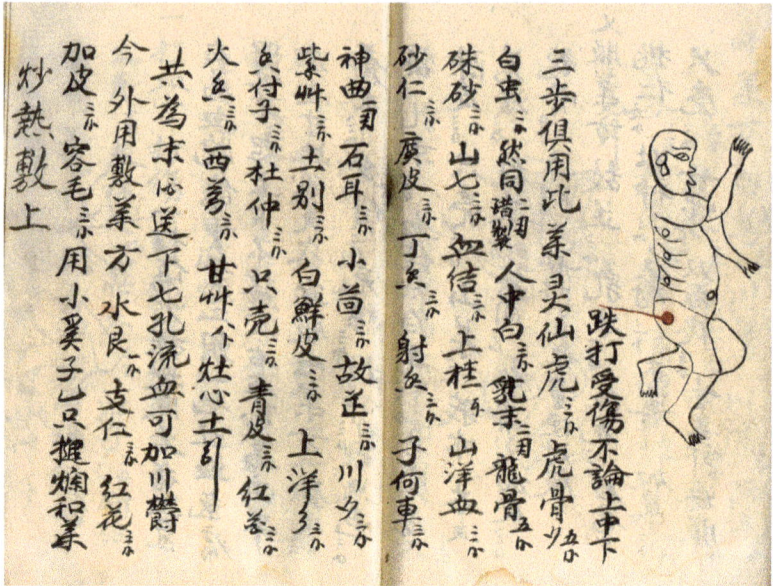

SURVEY OF CONTENTS: This is an example of writings on traumatology as they were widely distributed among the general population. Its contents are rather comprehensive. The initial paragraphs include Fen zuo you yao xing 分左右藥性, Fan die da quan shen yin jing yao 凡跌打全身引經藥 (in verses), Die da jie gu fu yao fang 跌打接骨敷藥方 (41 single substance recipes and fixed formulae).

Following a paragraph Fan die da sun shang yao xing 凡跌打損傷藥惟, a section explains that "man has 18 big holes, and 36 small holes", 人有十八大穴，三十六小穴, which are then discussed one after another with advice for pharmaceutical therapy. Next is a "table of contents", mu lu 目錄, listing paragraphs on 石傷太陽天庭鳳羽名盆弦, 兩膊名童骨, 牙腮掛膀心窩名天平針, 耳叢耳傍名左右下, 肚角背滿將臺脊下名雙蛇入洞, 米結舌腌名銅壺滴漏, 血腕下名淨瓶, 刀傷嬌空上中下背脊名頂樑, 膝腌, 對口, 肚臍, 腰下, 脅名血路, 咽喉, 命宮, 項圈乳傍名二仙傳道　中腕, 下竅. The following text, though, does not follow this "table of contents" but has its own structure. In general, an injury is shown by a drawing with a brief description and an advice on which pharmaceutical recipe to apply.

The rich contents of this volume do not allow to prepare a complete survey here. A counting of the pharmaceutical recipes finds approximately 160 formulae. They include the following recipe to achieve anesthesia: "sheng na cao 生拏草, chuan nan xing 川南星, sheng ban xia 生半夏, fan jiao 番椒, nao yang hua 鬧陽花, cao wu zi 草烏子. These ingredients are to be powderized together.

Each dosis: 1 *qian* 錢. One must not ingest much!" Such recipes were commonly used by the people.

***

| | |
|---|---|
| TITLE: | *Shang ke ji shu* 傷科集書, Collection of writings on traumatology |
| ID: | 8924 |
| CONTENTS: | Bone setting, traumatology |
| APPEARANCE: | Large format ancient manuscript volume. Cover made of thick kraft paper. No title label. Personal seal: 鄺？橋. Writing by numerous different hands. Calligraphy uneven, at times excellent, at times inferior. |
| BINDING: | Paper spills |
| MEASURE: | 27.2 x 17.8 |
| TITLE PAGE: | No |
| NO. OF PAGES: | 76 |
| L.P. /CH.L: | Mostly 9 x 23. Irregular. Smaller and larger characters, interspersed with drawings. |

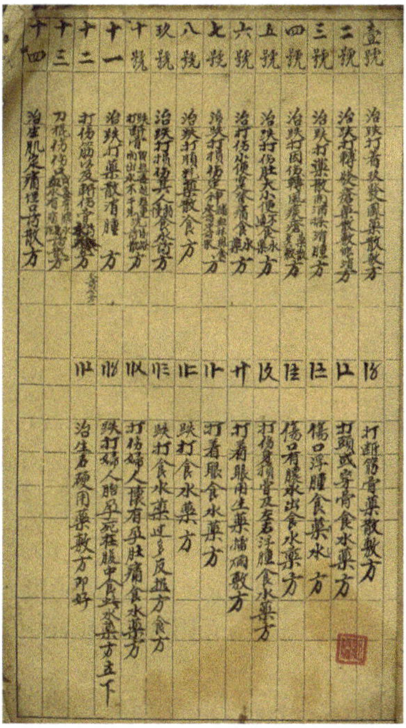

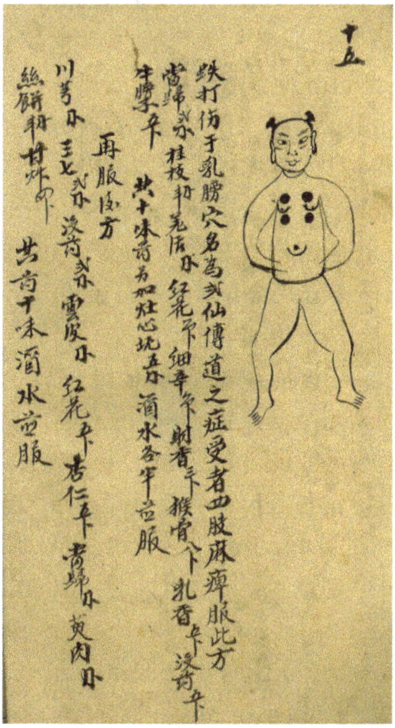

LAYOUT:          Written on printed account book paper but without adher-
                 ence to its line structures.
AUTHOR AND YEAR OF TEXT:
                 Unknown
YEAR OF COPY:    Date provided in the text: 31st year Republican era, i.e., 1942.

SURVEY OF CONTENTS: This volume focusses on bonesetting and traumatology. However it was neither copied from one single book, nor written by one
person. Its contents can be divided into the following sections.

1. Recipes to treat injuries resulting from falls and blows. This section begins
   with a table of contents listing and enumerating 26 recipes. The names
   of the recipes are quite detailed, for example: 治跌打著玖發風藥散敷方,
   "recipe for a powder medication applied externally to release wind to cure
   [injuries resulting from] falls and blows that have lasted for long." All other
   titles are of this type. Following the table of contents all 26 recipes are
   documented, with their structures, amounts of ingredients, and mode of
   application.

2. Recipes of Chen Xianlao 岑顯榮方. An introductory remark states: 此八藥
   方班中岑顯榮抄出經送經驗如神, "these eight pharmaceutical recipes have
   been hand-copied by Banzhong Chen Xianlao, were given away to others,
   and have proven to be divinely effective."

3. 班中跌打童人脈門部位全科, "Banzhong's complete medical specialty of
   [treating injuries of] boys [resulting from] falls and blows". This section has
   only 1 page. Above an inscription states: 由民國卅一年歲次壬午李顯經的
   筆抄/班中跌打童人脈門部位全科/傷著藥方列明一看便知. This section
   constitutes one of the main parts of the entire volume. It comprises 34
   paragraphs. Each paragraph includes a drawing to point out the location of
   an injury, with notes on its prognosis and the pharmaceutical recipes to be
   used for its therapy.

4. This is a long discourse of 1624 characters on bone injuries. It begins with
   a statement 傷頂門破骨入肉者，難治必死..., "Injuries caused to the top
   of the skull, breaking the bones and entering the flesh are hard to cure and
   will inevitably result in death." The final statement is on ...丹田受傷，臍下
   一寸二分, "injuries received by the cinnabar field, 1,2 inches below the navel". This section discusses the different causes and pathological conditions
   of injuries received at the various body parts, and the appropriate therapeutic approaches. The contents are abundant.

5. 33 Recipes for miscellaneous conditions. The heading states: 白濁鵝腮瘡

驗方, "Proven recipes for white and turbid goose cheek and *gan*-illness".
A later heading is: 肚腫腳腫五腫全方, "A complete [list of] recipes for
abdominal swelling, swollen legs, and the further five types of swelling". The
therapeutic indications range from venereal disease, *hua liu bing* 花柳病, to
swelling. They are not related to traumatology.

6. "Recipes transmitted by Feng Dexing", Feng Dexing chuan fang 馮得星傳方.
   The initial line states: 鶴山縣人馮得星先生祖傳下秘全跌打良方, "Mr. Feng
   Dexing's of He shan xian good recipes for [injuries from] falls and blows
   handed down in the family and kept secret as a whole". The recipes are
   divided into those to be applied for injuries of the upper, middle, and lower
   sections of the body. They are followed by further 36 recipes based on the
   experience of Feng Dexing, as well as other recipes to be applied in traumatology.

7. Miscellaneous recipes of diverse nature from 花柳埋小丸方, "a recipe for
   small pills to be prepared for sexually transmitted diseases", to the final indication 五臟辨症, "Different pathological signs of the five types of dropsy
   swelling". Recipes for "*gu*-swelling", *gu zhang* 蠱脹, are particularly numerous. These cases of "*gu*-swelling" may have been caused by hookworm
   disease or fluke disease prevalent in South China.

The terminology used, the pharmaceutical substances recommended, and
place names mentioned suggest that this is a folk text originating from Guang-
dong. Its contents are quite rich; it is very valuable.

*** 

| | |
|---|---|
| TITLE: | (*Xiao er tui na shu* 小兒推拿書, Book on pediatric push-and-pull massage) |
| ID: | 8925 |
| CONTENTS: | Pediatrics |
| APPEARANCE: | Ancient manuscript volume. Cover and front page without title. Orderly calligraphy. |
| BINDING: | Thread |
| MEASURE: | 19.4 x 14.3 |
| TITLE PAGE: | No |
| NO. OF PAGES: | 25 |
| L.P. /CH.L: | 8 x 20. Characters in the margins small and up to 13 columns per page. |

LAYOUT:                No lines, no frames. Numerous comments inserted in the
                       top margins.
AUTHOR AND YEAR OF TEXT:
                       Anonymous, Qing era.
YEAR OF COPY:   Character 玄 written with final stroke omitted. Late Qing
                       dynasty.

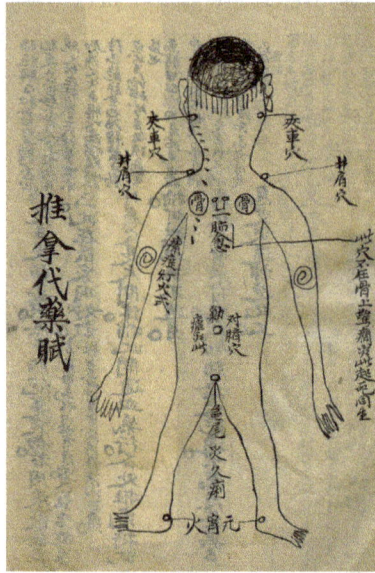

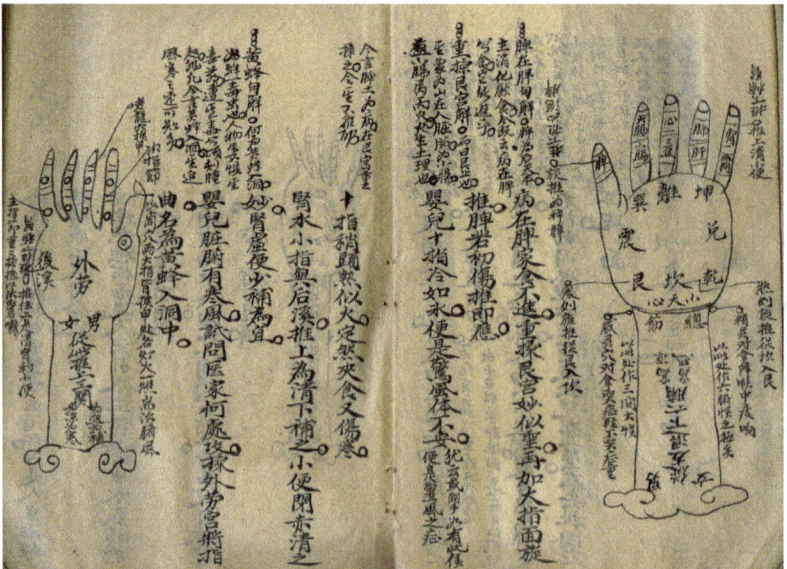

SURVEY OF CONTENTS: The first 2 ½ pages of this volume are not related to health care. They document poems.

Beginning with the third page the volume focusses on pediatric push-and-pull massage (*tui na* 推拿); it includes drawings and text (mostly written in rhymes) discussing pathological conditions suitable for *tui na* treatment. For the time being it remains unclear from which printed book the current volume was copied. The text repeatedly quotes verses from the Qing author Xia Ding's 夏鼎 (Yuzhu 禹鑄) *You ke tie jing* 幼科鐵鏡, "Iron Mirror of Pediatrics", printed in 1695. For example, the present volume's paragraph Tui na yi shi ge 推拿宜時歌 is in fact an excerpt from the *You ke tie jing*'s 幼科鐵鏡 paragraph Zhuo xi jia chuan kou jue 卓溪家傳口訣. The paragraph Wang yan se shen miao qiao zhi biao li han re xu shi ge 望顏色審苗竅知表裡寒熱虛實歌, "Song on inspecting complexion and examining the body openings to recognize [whether an illness is a case of] external or internal cold or heat, depletion or repletion", is identical with the *You ke tie jing*'s 幼科鐵鏡 paragraph Kan bing mi jue 看病秘訣, "Secret instructions on how to diagnose", with only the title changed. The paragraph Tui na dai yao fu 推拿代藥賦, "Poem on how to replace medication by push-and-pull massage", was quoted without modification from the *You ke tie jing* 幼科鐵鏡. However, we have not been able to trace the present volume's long discourse Xin cheng fu 心誠賦 to a possible source text.

*** 

| | |
|---|---|
| TITLE: | (*Yao fang. Ling yi shuo hua* 藥方·鈴醫說話. Pharmaceutical recipes. Sayings of itinerant physicians) |
| ID: | 8926 |
| CONTENTS: | Pharmaceutical recipes. Itinerant physicians. |
| APPEARANCE: | Ancient manuscript volume. Brittle paper quality. Edges and margins damaged. Calligraphy deficient. |
| BINDING: | Thread |
| MEASURE: | 24.3 x 13.1 |
| TITLE PAGE: | No |
| NO. OF PAGES: | 36 |
| L.P. /CH.L: | 8 x approx. 17 |
| LAYOUT: | No lines, no frames |
| AUTHOR AND YEAR OF TEXT: | |
| | Anonymous, Qing dynasty. |

YEAR OF COPY: Inscription at the conclusion of the volume: 丙午年冬季德
書一本. Hence this volume was written in 1906.

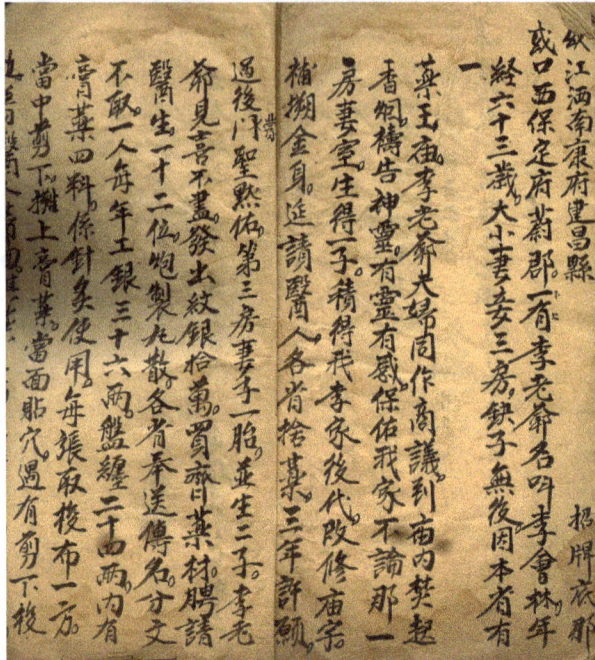

SURVEY OF CONTENTS: This volume has two major parts with different contents. The first part is a list of 73 pharmaceutical recipes. The latter part documents the rhetoric used by itinerant physicians to solicit customers.

The initial 25 pages list recipes that appear to have been casually recorded
over time as the author came to know of them; most are for common ailments.
This section further includes two paragraphs, Yao xing fu 藥性賦 and Yong yao
jie jing fu 用藥捷徑賦, "Poem on a short cut to the application of pharmaceutical therapy", that are partial copies of sections originally published by the
Ming author Luo Biwei 羅必煒 in his book Yi fang jie jing 醫方捷徑, "Short cut
to medical formulae".

The nine pages following page 26 are a record of statements made by itinerant physicians to "rope in" customers. In this section the author wrote down
theoretical passages as well as rhetoric phrases. These contents are reminis-
cent of those documented in the ms. 48041, Yi long zhi hu 醫龍治虎. An example is the following statement presumably prepared for use in a situation
where one onlooker may have said something to discourage someone else to
be treated by an itinerant healer: 有那一種二不流子光棍，把嘴一喇，他說

賣藥算卦，全憑說話。我（旧）〔就是〕重生的（蘆）〔盧〕醫，再世藥王，不言不語，（旧）〔誰〕知道, "There is that unmarried scoundrel saying such nonsense as 'to sell medication and to tell one's fortune, relies on rhetoric and nothing else'. Now, if I were the [famous ancient] Physician from Lu, or if I were the King of Medications reborn and would not speak, who would know [of my abilities]?"

Although the present text has many writing errors, it may still serve to confirm the widespread circulation of the contents of other such manuscripts, as for example, the *Yi long zhi hu* 醫龍治虎.

\*\*\*

| | |
|---|---|
| TITLE: | (*Yan ke ying yan liang fang* 眼科应验良方, Proven, good recipes in ophthalmology) |
| ID: | 8927 |
| CONTENTS: | Ophthalmology |
| APPEARANCE: | Ancient manuscript volume. Cover and first few pages lost. Calligraphy above average. |
| BINDING: | Thread |
| MEASURE: | 26.0 x 13.4 |

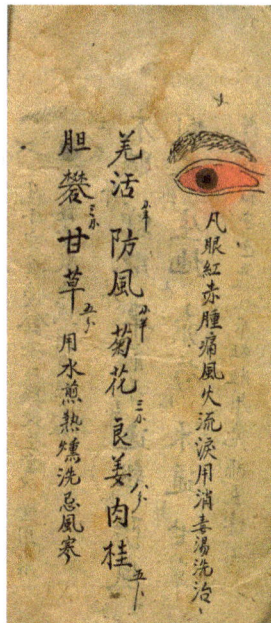

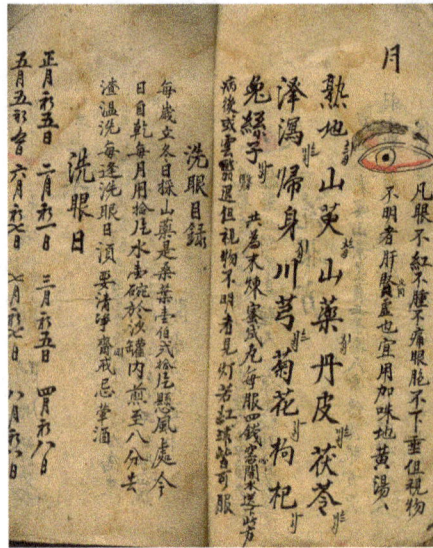

| TITLE PAGE: | No |
| --- | --- |
| NO. OF PAGES: | 20 |
| L.P. /CH.L: | 6-8 x approx. 20 |
| LAYOUT: | No lines, no frames |
| AUTHOR AND YEAR OF TEXT: | Cheng Songya 程松崖; Ming dynasty. |
| YEAR OF COPY: | The quality of the paper suggests that this volume was written in the Republican era. |

SURVEY OF CONTENTS: The contents are mostly focussed on ophthalmology. Each section begins with a drawing of an eye, with a few of these drawings indicating pathological changes by means of red ink. These drawings are followed by an explanatory text and pharmaceutical recipes. The fragmentary contents of this volume include 17 such sections. They include no hints at the identification of eye sectors in accordance with the Five Phases theory. The source text is the Ming author Cheng Songya's 程松崖 *Yan ke ying yan liang fang* 眼科应验良方, which was published in the *dao guang* 道光 reign period under the name of Ye Tianshi 葉天士. It was copied very often.

Following the illustrated section, the author recorded various ophthalmological recipes and advices, such as Xi yan mu lu 洗眼目錄, Xi yan ri 洗眼日, Tu si zi wan fang 菟絲子丸方, Xiao lu san 硝爐散, Xi yan zuo yang er ji lan zhe fang 洗眼作癢而及爛者方, and Tui hui pi yan liang fang 退灰皮眼良方.

This is followed by a section beginning with a title Zhi xiao er ke chu 治小兒科處, "Formulae treatments in pediatrics", documenting 17 recipes for various ailments from the realms of pediatrics, gynecology, and internal medicine. The author also recorded recipes that are not related to medicine, such as *shui dou zhi fang* 水豆豉方, "recipe for fermented soy beans kept in water", and *bian dan fang* 變蛋方, "recipe for modifying eggs", the latter detailing how to prepare *pi dan* 皮蛋, "preserved eggs":

The volume ends with sections Da hun bu he zhun ge 大婚不合準歌, "Song on incompatibilities [of possible partners] in a marriage", and Qu xi fu ji shu da dao xing 娶媳婦忌屬大道行, "Grand competence in what is to be avoided when taking a wife", reflecting marriage customs of the time.

\*\*\*

| | |
|---|---|
| TITLE: | *Hou ke mi yue* 喉科秘籥, a secret key to laryngology. |
| ID: | 8928 |
| CONTENTS: | Laryngology |
| APPEARANCE: | Poor, thin ancient manuscript volume. Cover with inscription: 喉科秘籥. Lower right, small rectangular seal: 廷珍. Good calligraphy. |
| BINDING: | Thread |
| MEASURE: | 17.0 x 12.9 |
| TITLE PAGE: | No |

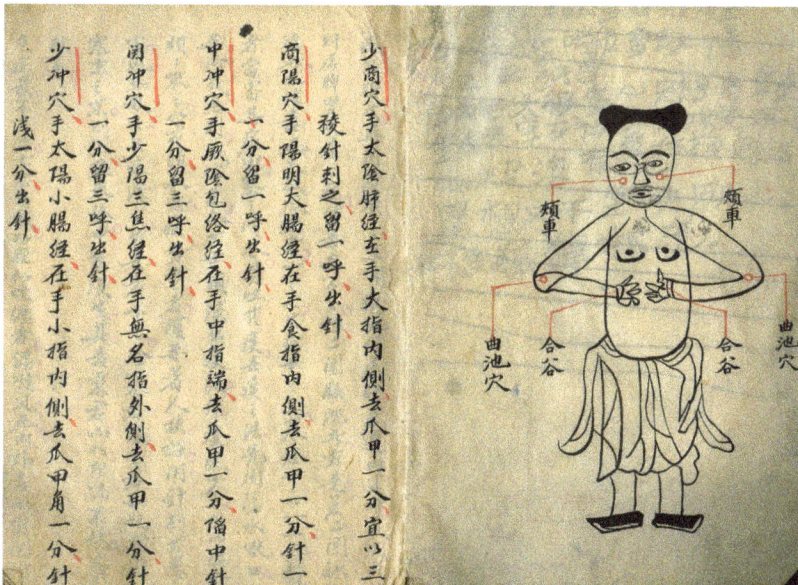

NO. OF PAGES:        14
L.P. /CH.L:          10 x 27
LAYOUT:              No lines, no frames
AUTHOR AND YEAR OF TEXT:     Zheng Chen 鄭塵; Amended by Xu Zuoting
                     許佐廷. 19th century.
YEAR OF COPY:    Not clearly identifiable. Perhaps late Qing early Republican
                     era.

SURVEY OF CONTENTS: This is a text on laryngology. The inscription *Hou ke mi yue* 喉科秘籥 on the cover refers to a book written, during the Qing dynasty, by Zheng Chen 鄭塵, a descendant of Zheng Meijian 鄭梅潤, which was revised and enlarged later by Xu Zuoting 許佐廷. The focus of the text is on *bai chan hou* 白纏候, "signs of white twining", i.e., diphtheria. The present volume is only a partical excerpt. On its first page it shows a human figure indicating the locations of three acupuncture holes on the left and on the right. The opposite page lists five further acupuncture points, and identifies their locations, and informs of how deep a needle may be inserted there and for what time it should be left in the tissue before it is withdrawn again. The back of this page, i.e., its second half, is missing, and with it the beginning of the text. The same is true further on in the volume; individual pages have been torn out, leaving gaps in the continuation of the text. Generally speaking, different laryngological conditions are discussed, with appropriate pharmaceutical and acupuncture therapies. Some of the paragraphs are rhymed. Towards the end, a paragraph has the title Hou zheng bu bian bai chan hou feng lun 喉證補編白纏喉風論. It includes a line: "偶閲家傳手錄，于乾隆五十年，旱荒秋見者症，其傳染生死光景如前，名曰白纏喉……" This is evidence that the text was copied from Zheng Chen's book.

***

TITLE:           (*Kan dou fa* 看痘法, Patterns of diagnosing smallpox)
ID:              8929
CONTENTS:        Smallpox
APPEARANCE:      Ancient manuscript volume. Edges, margins damaged. Average calligraphy. Cover stained, prepared from various layers of cotton paper glued together. Top left segment missing. Only lower most character of title inscription left

readable: 論. Back of front cover with inscription: 彭學英.
Also, inscription there, written with fountain pen: 彭學英
計，諸人不借。後人善管，萬勿遺失，開卷便知. At the
beginning of the text, a seal without frame: 王光有記. Back
cover inside, inscription written with red ink: 汪純五置/乙
亥.

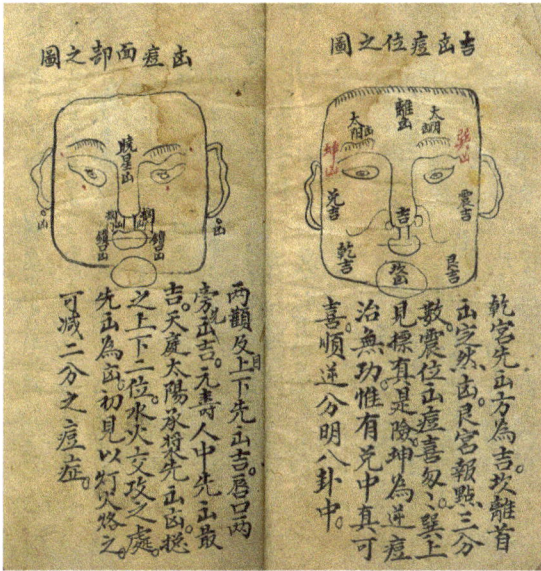

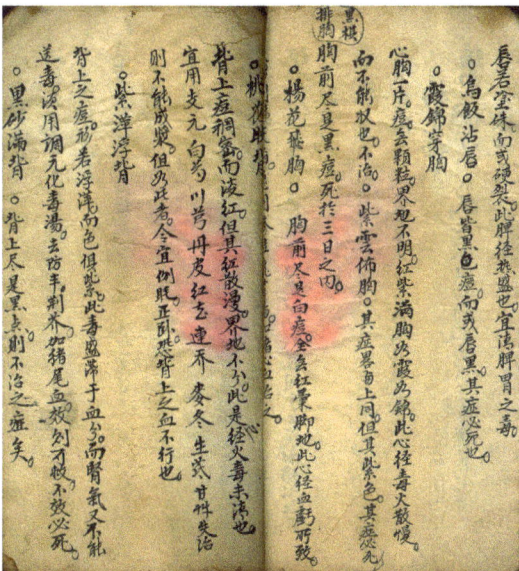

BINDING:          Thread
MEASURE:          21.1 x 12.3
TITLE PAGE:       No
NO. OF PAGES:     33
L.P. /CH.L:       8 x 24
LAYOUT:           No lines, no frames
AUTHOR AND YEAR OF TEXT:
                  Unknown
YEAR OF COPY:     No taboos observed. Republican era.

SURVEY OF CONTENTS: This is a text on smallpox. The initial paragraphs have
the following titles: 治臍風藥方, "Pharmaceutical recipes for navel wind", 搽
藥方"Recipes for ointments", 臍風驚, "Navel wind fright", 歷代藥王脈師主, a
listing of "Medicine Kings of 13 generations", ending with an apotropaic incantation. Apparently, these paragraphs originate from a different source than the
following contents of the present volume.

The main text begins with a paragraph: Kan dou jin fa 看痘筋法. The titles
of the following paragraphs are: 論痘發日期、痘症日期、摘痘法、將燃照
法、面分八卦之圖 (with a drawing of the human face)、五臟面位之圖 (with
a drawing of the human face)、吉凶痘位之圖 (with a drawing of the human
face)、兇痘面部之圖 (with a drawing of the human face)、看痘後舌法、看
兇痘秘訣、見點認痘法、夾水痘、疔痘、入門認異痘、天根痘、天空痘、
蝕痘、海溢痘、海枯痘、有根痘、抱鼻痘、單鎖口雙鎖口、鎖頂托頤、豬
頸痘、足痘、鬼摸痘、鬼痘、賊痘、蛇皮痘、藥患痘、九焦痘、伏陰痘、
空瘖痘、石白痘、茱萸痘、蟲痘、血泡痘、血靨痘、口痘、口痘、口痘、琉
璃痘、赤萍紫萍白萍痘、黑痘、氣血兩敗痘、復出痘。A subsequent sec-
tion, "Master of the Cloud Wing's 28 types of irregular appearances of pox",
Yun yi zi er shi ba ban guai dou 雲翼子二十八般怪痘, lists the following ab-
normal   conditions:   丹雲繞頂、紫雲貫頂、烏紗覆頂、黎花幔頂、雲掩天
庭、紫萍鋪額、烏紗蓋額、灰撲印堂、紅紗拂面、楊花拂面、赤硃繞唇、
烏飯沾唇、霞錦穿胸、楊花飛胸、桃花映背、紫萍浮背、黑砂滿背、雲鋪
魚背、赤鱗穿腹、黑蝦纏腹、白黎落地、葡萄落地、爛栗居臀、榴花遍
野、黑珠遍體、楊花發枝。

Next is a section Er shi si ding fang 二十四頂方, "24 top recipes", informing
of the appearances of pox erupting at different times, and the appropriate recipes to be applied for their therapy, and a further section Zhi dou yao fang 治痘
藥方, "pharmaceutical recipes for curing pox".

The volume ends with a list of further 39 recipes, such as *fa biao jie du tang* 發表解毒湯, "decoction to resolve the exterior to dissolve poison", *shen qin bai zhu san* 參苓白朮散, "powder with *shen*, *qin* and *bai zhu*", *nei tuo san* 內托散, "powder for internal support", and *qing jin san* 清金散, "powder to clear metal (i.e., the lung)".

Many of the names recorded here for specific conditions of smallpox are not known from any other text. They may evidence an early or only locally available understanding of the disease and its different manifestations. Further research may reveal their origin, and further sources where they are used.

*** 

| | |
|---|---|
| TITLE: | (*Yan hou si shi ba zheng* 咽喉四十八症, Forty eight pathological conditions of guts and throat) |
| ID: | 8930 |
| CONTENTS: | Laryngology |
| APPEARANCE: | Ancient manuscript volume. Paper aged. Cover added by later hand. No title. Careful handwriting. Average calligraphy. |
| BINDING: | Thread |
| MEASURE: | 20.6 x 14.4 |
| TITLE PAGE: | No |
| NO. OF PAGES: | 21 |
| L.P. /CH.L: | 12 x 22 |
| LAYOUT: | No lines, no frames |
| AUTHOR AND YEAR OF TEXT: | |
| | Anonymous, Qing. |
| YEAR OF COPY: | No taboos observed. Republican era. |

SURVEY OF CONTENTS: This is a book on laryngology with very special contents. The very first line of the text has the heading 治咽喉四十捌症外加式症予, with the final character erroneously used for: 序. No author's name is given.

Following this long initial discourse is a table of contents listing 48 pathological conditions: 纏喉風、鎖喉風、上顎懸（風）〔癰〕、單乳蛾、氣丹、左右丁瘡、【口秦】舌〔瘡〕、左右雀舌、纏舌喉風、雙單活乳蛾、重舌、雙單死乳蛾、走馬喉風、走馬牙疳、喉痹、梅核氣、喉疳瘡、迎舌癰、小兒珍珠瘡、大小人一切珍珠瘡、舌上紅癤、欠舌喉風、死乳蛾核、開花疔、寒後生（痰）〔疾〕、蟲蝕喉瘡、舌下蓮花、蝼蟻氣丹、兜腮癤、汗後生癰、左陽瘡、右陰瘡、舌癰、舌丁生瘡、重顎風、帝中風、松子風、魚鱗瘡、燕口風、咽喉風、蟻喉風、懸旗風、架角風、搜牙風、風牙癰、上顎癰、上下左右牙齒.

This table of contents is followed by a lengthy paragraph discussing various forms of such ailments with their appropriate treatment, but without specifying the constituents of the pharmaceutical recipes mentioned. Next are two stories of historical experts in laryngology, first, a person from Jiang xi 江夏 with the name Wang Tianchong 王天寵, another from the *wan li* 萬曆 reign period, by Yin Huiyan 印惠琰 of Yu shan 玉山 in Jiang xi 江西.

This is followed by 26 recipes for use in laryngology, including one anesthesia recipe with the following ingredients: *chuan wu* 川烏, *cao wu* 草烏, *huai wu* 淮烏, *xi xin* 細辛, *yuan cun* 原寸, and *bing pian* 冰片 to be ground to powder and blown into the nose.

Next is the main body of this book, a listing of 48 laryngological conditions, each with a drawing and an explanatory text, as well as advice for treatment with needles and pharmaceutical recipes. The text ends with the section *Han hou sheng ji* 寒後生疾, "ailments following a cold". The remaining 21 conditions listed in the initial table of contents are missing. Hence this is only a fragment. The text does not mention diphtheria, which indicates that the text dated from before the *qian long* 乾隆 reign period. The way the pathological conditions are identified is quite peculiar. Treatments include both internal and external approaches.

***

| | |
|---|---|
| TITLE: | *Shang han wen yi she tai* 傷寒瘟疫舌胎, Tongue coating in the case of harm caused by cold and warmth epidemics. |
| ID: | 8931 |
| CONTENTS: | Tongue diagnosis |
| APPEARANCE: | Ancient manuscript volume of poor appearance. Cover with inscription, upper left: 傷寒瘟疫舌胎一共全部. Lower right: 張旺生記. Ink and calligraphy differ from title, added by later hand. Center, a date 乙卯年, plus a recipe for syphilis. Main text with average calligraphy. |
| BINDING: | Paper spills |
| MEASURE: | 21.0 x 11.5 |
| TITLE PAGE: | No |
| NO. OF PAGES: | 13 |
| L.P. /CH.L: | 6-8 x. 22 |
| LAYOUT: | No lines, no frames |

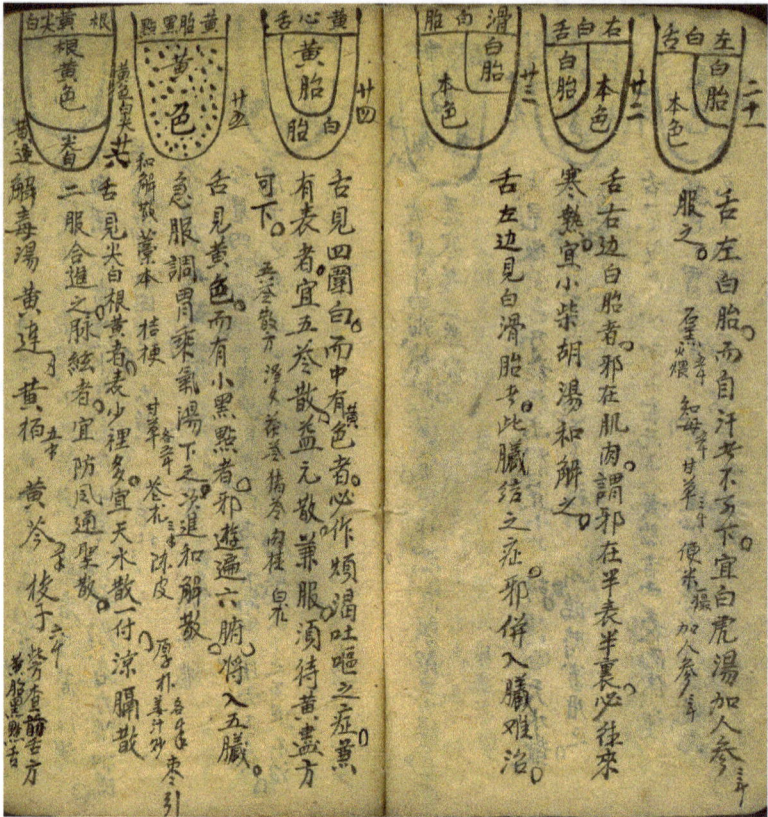

AUTHOR AND YEAR OF TEXT:

Mr. Ao 敖氏, Yuan, 1341.

YEAR OF COPY:    No taboos observed. Republican era.

SURVEY OF CONTENTS: The use of the term 胎 in the title indicates that the source text of this volume dates from prior to the mid-Qing dynasty. The text has neither preface nor table of contents. From the beginning it lists 36 different variations of tongue coating, with a drawing and an explanatory text. A comparison shows that this is a copy of the *Ao shi shang han jin jing lu* 敖氏傷寒金鏡錄, "Mr. Ao's Golden Mirror of Harm Caused by Cold". However, in the present copy the sequence of the 36 tongue conditions was modified, and this applies also to a small number of wordings in the text.

The final pages of this volume list a dozen or so pharmaceutical recipes.

***

TITLE: *Hei shen wan yao fang* 黑神丸藥方, Black spirits pills, a pharmaceutical recipe

ID: 8932

CONTENTS: Pharmaceutical recipe

APPEARANCE: Ancient manuscript volume of better than average quality. Cover with inscription: 黑神丸藥方壹部/瑞記/庚寅年臘錄. At the beginning of the main text, small rectangular seal, characters cut in relief: 王藏鼎章.

BINDING: Thread

MEASURE: 20.8 x 13.7

TITLE PAGE: No

NO. OF PAGES: 16

L.P. /CH.L: 7 x 18- 21

LAYOUT: No lines, no frames

AUTHOR AND YEAR OF TEXT:

Unknown. Copyist's name: Rui 瑞

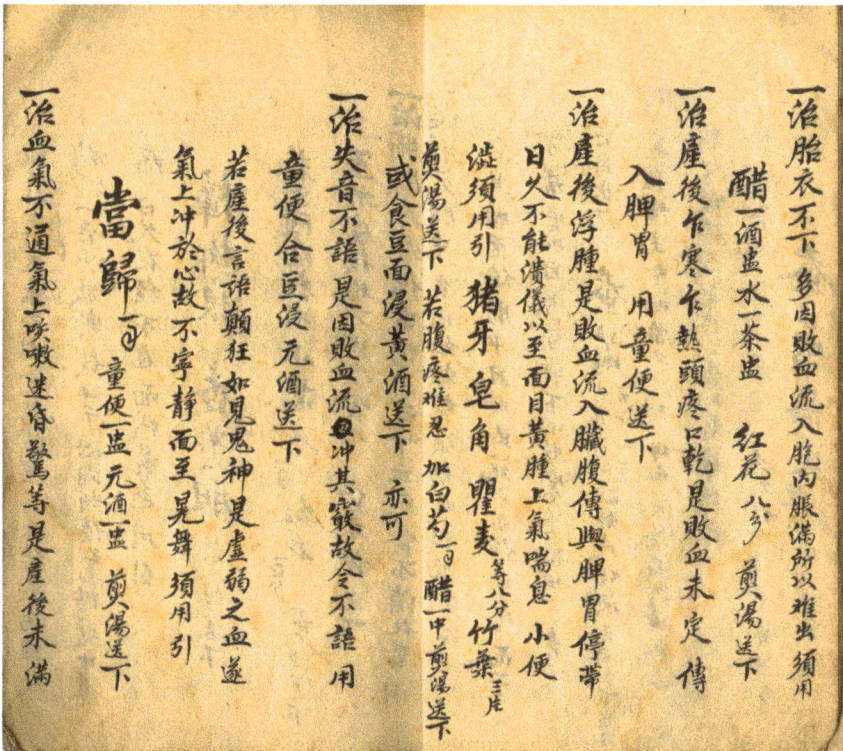

YEAR OF COPY:    The inscription on the cover, 庚寅年謄錄, suggests that this manuscript was written in either 1890 or 1950.

SURVEY OF CONTENTS: The first line of the main text says: 黒神丸方, followed by a list of the ingredients of this recipe: 當歸、木香、明天麻、百草霜、飛羅麵、藏紅花、京墨. This is followed by a list of conditions for which an application of the Black Spirit Pills is advised, each with a modification of the recipe. The number of such conditions recorded here, 36, is smaller than in other such volumes where mostly 72 conditions are listed. The final two pages of the main text list a similar "cure all" formula, the "Black Gold Pills", *wu jin wan* 烏金丸. However the formula is not followed by a list of conditions requesting modified applications.

The use of a basic recipe for pills, and the modification of its ingredients, as well as the changing nature of liquids suggested to accompany ingestion for large numbers of gynecological ailments was very prevalent during the Qing dynasty. Hence copies of such texts were often prepared and widely distributed among the people.

***

TITLE:          *Ti yong shuo yao lun* 體用說藥論, On medication explained on the basis of personal experience
ID:             8933
CONTENTS:       Therapeutic principles
APPEARANCE:     Ancient manuscript volume. Margins/edges severely damaged. Cover with stains, and two lines of inscription, vertical from left to right. 亢則害承乃制體用說藥論有五法/五運六氣風熱濕火燥寒/薛潤埴/高蓋先. The final three characters written with fountain pen by later hand. Copyist unknown. Two collectors/owners: Xue Runzhi 薛潤埴 and Gao Gaixian 高蓋先. Careful handwriting and calligraphy.
BINDING:        Thread
MEASURE:        19.6 x 10.7
TITLE PAGE:     No
NO. OF PAGES:   19
L.P. /CH.L:     6 x 21
LAYOUT:         No lines, no frames

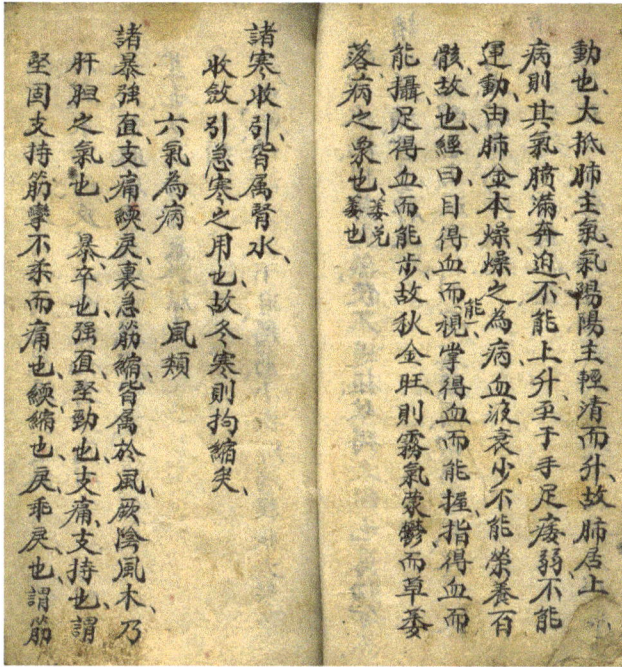

AUTHOR AND YEAR OF TEXT:

Unknown, possibly Qing dynasty.

YEAR OF COPY: Character 玄 at times written with final stroke omitted, at times written without observing the Qing era taboo. End of Qing/early Republican era.

SURVEY OF CONTENTS: Folk manuscripts only rarely discuss therapeutic principles. The present volume is an exception. The first paragraph is on Five Periods and Six Qi, *wu yun liu qi* 五運六氣, and offers an introduction to the basic concepts of this theory. Next is a discourse Wu yun zhu bing 五運主病, with 19 paragraphs on illness dynamics, briefly naming pathological conditions and their underlying dynamics. For example, Zhu feng diao xuan jie shu gan mu 諸風掉眩, 皆屬肝木, "All types of wind, with shaking and dizziness, they belong to the liver and wood." And: Zhu tong yang chuang yang jie shu xin huo 諸痛癢瘡瘍, 皆屬心火, "All types of pain, itch, sores and ulcers, they belong to the heart and fire." The next section is on *feng lei* 風類, "Types of wind", and *re lei* 熱類, "Types of heat". The rest is missing.

***

| | |
|---|---|
| TITLE: | *Fu ying zhi zhang tui na qi yao* 福嬰指掌推拿輯要, Essentials of push-and-pull massage as a guide for happy children |
| ID: | 8934 |
| CONTENTS: | Pediatrics |
| APPEARANCE: | Ancient manuscript volume. Cover stained and partly worn. Inscription: 福嬰指掌推拿輯要/豐慶堂記. Edges with some minor damage, but text complete. Good calligraphy. Handwriting disorderly. Table of contents. |
| BINDING: | Thread |
| MEASURE: | 14.5 x 22.6 |
| TITLE PAGE: | Yes, with inscription: 福嬰指掌/王廷祿記/癸巳製. |
| NO. OF PAGES: | 42 |
| L.P. /CH.L: | 16 x 13 |
| LAYOUT: | No lines, no frames |
| AUTHOR AND YEAR OF TEXT: | |
| | Qing, Zhou Songling 周松齡. |
| YEAR OF COPY: | The manuscript is dated "produced in [the year] *gui si*" 癸巳製. This could be 1893 and sixty years later 1953. The way of handwriting and the quality of the paper may suggest that this copy dates from 1953, but this is not certain. |

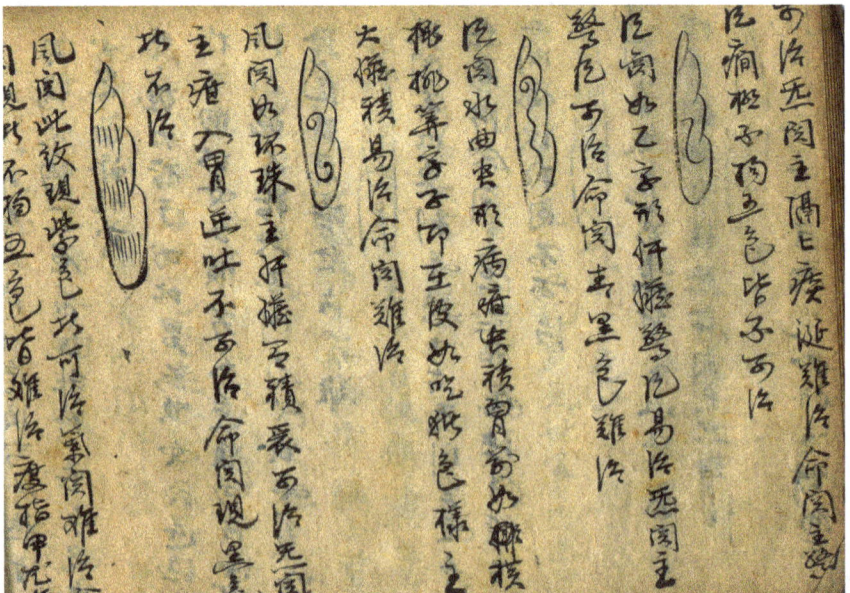

SURVEY OF CONTENTS: The title of this volume given on the cover is *Fu ying zhi zhang* 福嬰指掌, "Guide to happy infants". The "table of contents" at the beginning lists a "Preface to the *Tui na qi yao* 推拿輯要", and its three *juan*. The Preface to the *Tui na qi yao* 推拿輯要 was signed: 道光癸卯東黃增生周松齡仙渠氏序. It informs that father and son studied the *Fu ying zhi zhang* 福嬰指掌 written in the year *ren xu* 壬戌 of the *jia qing* 嘉慶 reign period by Li Qin 李芹, and then took up *tui na* 推拿 push-and-pull massage for a living. Their own book was printed, and is recorded in the *Zhong guo zhong yi gu ji zong mu* 中國中醫古籍總目, as *Xiao er tui na qi yao* 小兒推拿輯要, by the Qing author Zhou Songling 周松齡, (Xianqu 仙渠, Jiayan 家嚴). It was edited during the Republican period by Song Letian 宋樂天 (Wuhuai zi 無懷子). The book by the Zhous was completed in 1843; presently known to exist are lead print copies by An dong cheng wen xin shu ju 安東誠文信書局鉛印本 of 1933 and 1940. However, the present volume has no reference to the printing edited by Son Letian 宋樂天 during the Republican era.

According to its table of contents, the present volume should have three *juan*. However it has only the first two *juan*; *juan* 3 is missing. The first *juan* focusses on the diagnosis of children's diseases, mostly by visual inspection and by examining finger lines (the text includes 17 drawings of finger lines), and it also has some sections on the physiology and pathology of children. The second *juan* is devoted to the treatment of common pediatric illnesses by *tui na* 推拿 push-and-pull massage. It has no explanatory drawings, only text. The third *juan* is indicated in the table of contents as including drawings of the back of the hand and palm, i.e., Yang zhang tu 陽掌圖 and Yin zhang tu 陰掌圖, however since the 3rd *juan* is missing in this volume, their nature remains unknown.

\*\*\*

TITLE: (*Dou ke er shi si jing deng huao zhi fa* 痘科·二十四驚燈火治法, The specialty concerned with smallpox. Lamp wick cauterization therapy patterns for twenty four conditions of fright)

ID: 8935

CONTENTS: Pediatrics

APPEARANCE: Ancient manuscript volume of average quality. No cover. Outer edges preserved by black glue to prevent damage. Careful handwriting. Average calligraphy.

治驚風
用燈火
部位圖

急驚口吐白沫

急驚用灯火法

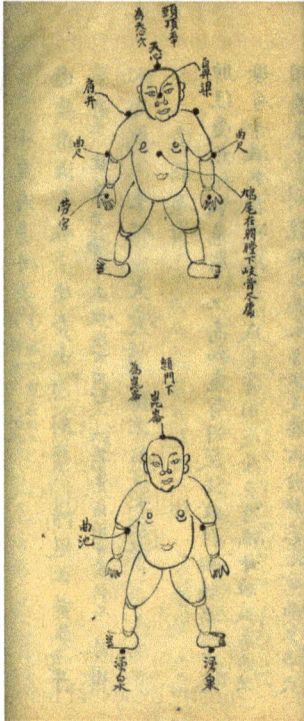

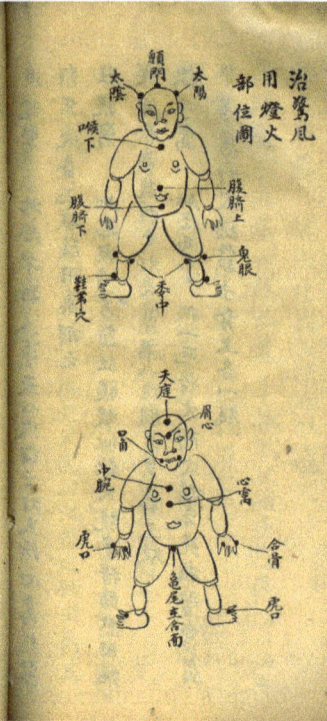

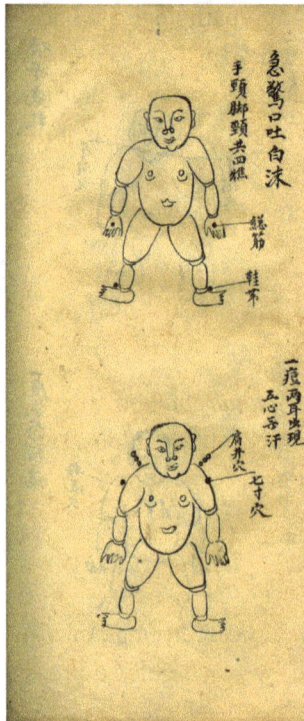

出瘟至一匕猶未見苗者名根地開花口乾舌生苫用
煨姜滿身擦遍熱水洗一次照各穴用火燋之令臥
覆被用白蠟手射氣三氣為末用缽一個將藥末入
缽內用鐵爺一柄燒紅酒一碗將酒淬爺酒溺入缽
中取服少許連缽放入被內取汗為度汗乾瘟出

BINDING:            Originally paper spills. Restored with thread binding.
MEASURE:            23.9 x 12.6
TITLE PAGE:         No
NO. OF PAGES:       66
L.P. /CH.L:         8 x 20
LAYOUT:             No lines, no frames
AUTHOR AND YEAR OF TEXT:
                    Unknown, Qing dynasty.
YEAR OF COPY:       The nature of the paper and the absence of characters writ-
                    ten to obey Qing dynasty taboos suggest that this manu-
                    script volume was written in the Republican era.


SURVEY OF CONTENTS: This volume was copied from two very rare pediatric
books.

The first is on smallpox. It has a table of contents, beginning with paragraphs
on 痘之源流論、痘疹辨、五臟合一解、解毒辨、認疗法 and ending with 化
癍散、痘科、痘後補劑末藥方. It also includes discourses on rhinozeros horn,
Xi jiao lun 犀角論, and on stag antlers: Lu rong lun 鹿茸論. No date or author
of this first source text are mentioned, but it quotes Zhu Chungu's 朱純詁 Dou
zhen ding *lun* 痘疹定論. This book is described as 治法頗屬詳備也，獨奈痘
眼、痘毒、痘痢三症毫無一驗, "The therapeutic methods are quite encompassing. Only the [treatments recommended for] the three disease conditions
ailments of the eyes associated with smallpox, smallpox poison, and diarrhea
associated with smallpox have no therapeutic effects whatsoever." Two further
texts are quoted that are not listed in any of the bibliographies known to us: Li
Juesi's 李覺斯 *Dou zhen lei bian* 痘疹類編, and Zhang Yi's 張熠, *Bao chi quan
shu* 保赤全書. The source text is yet to be identified.

The second book has no title either. It too provides a table of contents, start-
ing with the paragraphs 小兒科論、通治三法、小兒科方、萬全湯、感冒風
寒方、痢疾、瘧疾, and ending with 驚症、吐瀉、小兒肚臍突出半寸方. This
book's structure is rather disorderly. Its first half offers advice on the application of pharmaceutical recipes. The latter half focusses on the lamp wick
cauterization treatment of 24 fright conditions. There is also a paragraph devoted to "Lamp wick cauterization therapy patterns for the cure of smallpox."
32 drawings of the human body show the locations where lamp wick cauterization is to be applied.

\*\*\*

| | |
|---|---|
| TITLE: | (*Mai shu. Xiao er tui na* 脈書·小兒推拿, Scripture on Vessels. Pediatric *tuina* push-and-pull massage) |
| ID: | 8936 |
| CONTENTS: | Pulse diagnosis. Pediatrics. |
| APPEARANCE: | Ancient manuscript volume. Cover severely damaged. Inscription: 喬步陞/積善堂題. Final page(s?) missing. Main text complete. Careful handwriting. Good calligraphy. |
| BINDING: | Thread |
| MEASURE: | 18.5 x 12.6 |
| TITLE PAGE: | No |
| NO. OF PAGES: | 50 |
| L.P. /CH.L: | 10 x 25 |
| LAYOUT: | No lines, no frames |
| AUTHOR AND YEAR OF TEXT: | Unknown, Qing dynasty. Copy prepared by Qiao Busheng 喬步陞. |
| YEAR OF COPY: | Character 玄 not written to obey Qing dynasty taboo. Possibly Republican era. |

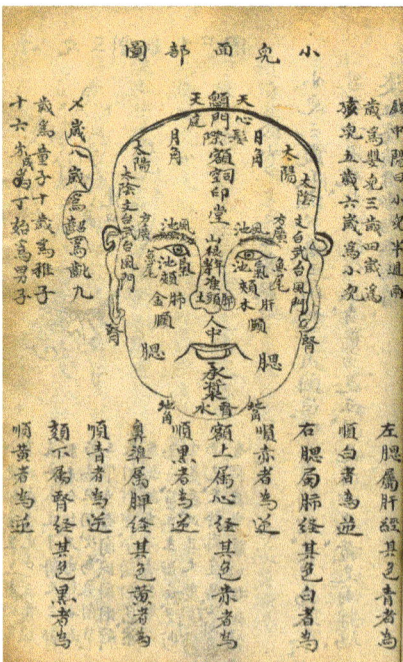

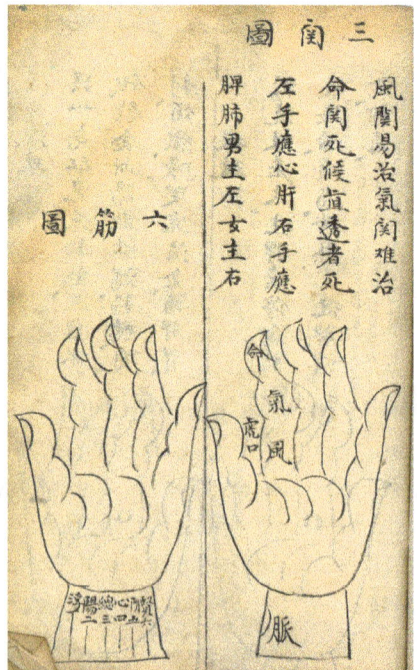

SURVEY OF CONTENTS: This volume was erroneously bound in that a page from the later section on *tui na* 推拿 massage became the first page. Beginning with its second page, this volume is devoted to pulse diagnosis. The headings of the various paragraphs are: 持脈手法、診脈三要、診家樞要、脈察六字、反關脈、脈貴有神、九候難調、男女異脈、老少異脈、心臟歌、肝臟歌、脾臟歌、肺臟歌、腎臟歌、診脈入式歌、孕婦傷寒歌、診産後傷寒脈歌. The text frequently quotes from the work on movements in the vessels written by Hua Boren 滑伯仁. The structure is of the type found in the *Mai jue* 脈訣.

This section is followed by a second part with a new title page, and a title given as follows: 針灸大成推掐揉等法/積善堂. The paragraphs bear the following titles: 手訣、保嬰神術、手法歌、觀形察色法、論色歌、認筋法歌、小兒面部圖, etc. The text includes ample advice on pediatric diagnosis, including visual examination and the examination of sections of the hands of patients, with paragraphs bearing titles such as 陽掌圖各穴手法仙訣, 陰掌圖各穴手法仙訣, 小兒用針, 小兒指紋三關圖, accompanied by more than 20 drawings of the entire human body, the human face, and finger lines. A subsequent section is devoted to pediatric nursing.

The final part bears the title "Rhymed instructions on manual disease therapy", Shou fa zhi bing jue 手法治病訣. This part records *tui na* 推拿 push-and-pull massage approaches, such as 黃蜂出洞、水底撈月、鳳單展翅, etc. This section is very unstructured. Its contents are not found in the *Zhen jiu da cheng* 針灸大成.

***

| | |
|---|---|
| TITLE: | (*Za chao ben* 雜抄本, Manuscript copy with various contents) |
| ID: | 8937 |
| CONTENTS: | Acupuncture, pharmaceutical recipes |
| APPEARANCE: | Ancient manuscript volume. Cover made of China blue paper. Cover and edges/margins with some damage. Average calligraphy. Handwriting casual. No title. |
| BINDING: | Thread |
| MEASURE: | 23.7 x 13.0 |
| TITLE PAGE: | Paper printed with red silk lines and frame. No inscription. |
| NO. OF PAGES: | 20 pp with medical-pharmaceutical contents. 7 pp. on fortune telling. 3 pp. with pharmaceutical recipes. 7 pp. on *ba zi* 八字 fortune telling. |

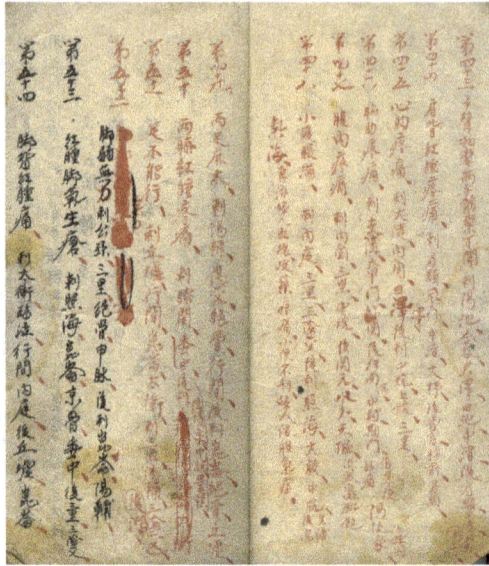

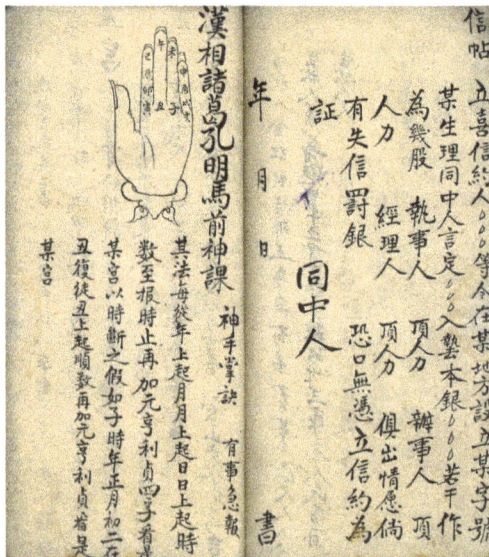

L.P. /CH.L:          7 x approx. 24
LAYOUT:              No lines, no frames
AUTHOR AND YEAR OF TEXT:
                     Unknown
YEAR OF COPY:        The character 玄 was not written to obey the Qing dynasty
                     taboo. This, and the quality of the paper suggest that this
                     volume dates from the Republican era.

SURVEY OF CONTENTS: The contents of this manuscript volume are quite mixed. Still, two major sections may be discerned: one on medical-pharmaceutical issues, the other one on fortune telling. The first two pages show one drawing each, first, "An illustration of facial moles of males", Nan ren mian zhi tu 男人面痣圖, and, second, "An illustration of facial moles of women", Nü ren mian zhi tu 女人面痣圖. Both are designed to predict a person's future by certain features in their face.

Beginning with the 3$^{rd}$ page, the volume focusses on acupuncture. The paragraphs are numbered, beginning from 5 and ending with 151. This is a list of as many pathological conditions and the insertion holes for a needle therapy. The text includes some Q & A dialogues to discuss the causes, pathological dynamics and appropriate therapy of illnesses. This section is followed by a list of 15 pharmaceutical recipes for illnesses such as cholera *huo luan* 霍亂, phlegm-fire *tan huo* 痰火, and malaria *nüe ji* 瘧疾.

Beginning with p. 21, the focus shifts to fortune telling, which is followed by another list of four pharmaceutical recipes. These are all fixed formulae copied from printed books. They include no folk recipes relying on one single ingredient.

*** 

| | |
|---|---|
| TITLE: | *Zeng bu zhu you shi san ke* 增補祝由十三科, Enlarged 13th specialty [of medicine] dealing with the invocation of the origins. |
| ID: | 8938 |
| CONTENTS: | Apotropaics |
| APPEARANCE: | This manuscript volume is enclosed in a golden cardboard case, added by a more recent owner who also glued a white paper slip on the outside with an inscription of deficient calligraphy: Zhu you ke chao ben 祝由科抄本, "Manuscript on the specialty of invocation of the origins". The volume's original cover and paper are cut from locally made 楮紙. paper of a rather crude quality. Careful handwriting. Average calligraphy. |
| BINDING: | Thread |
| MEASURE: | 21.8 x 11.0 |

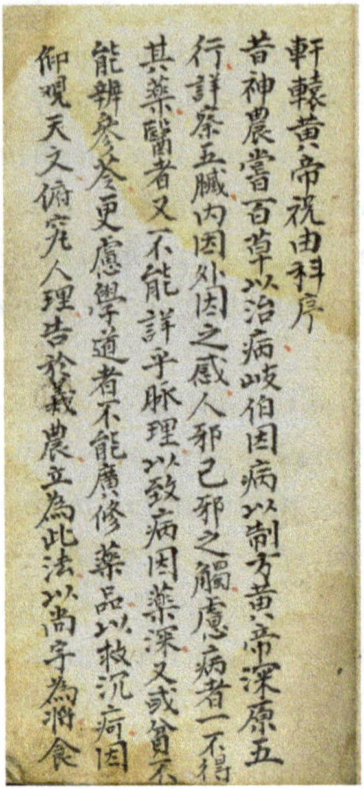

軒轅黃帝祝由科序
昔神農嘗百草以治病岐伯因病以制方黃帝深原五
行詳察五臓内因外困之感人邪己邪之觸慮病者一不得
其藥醫者又不能詳乎脉理以致病困藥深又或貧不
能辦參苓更慮學道者不能廣修藥品以救沉疴因
仰觀天文俯究人理告於栽農立為此法以尚字為湖食

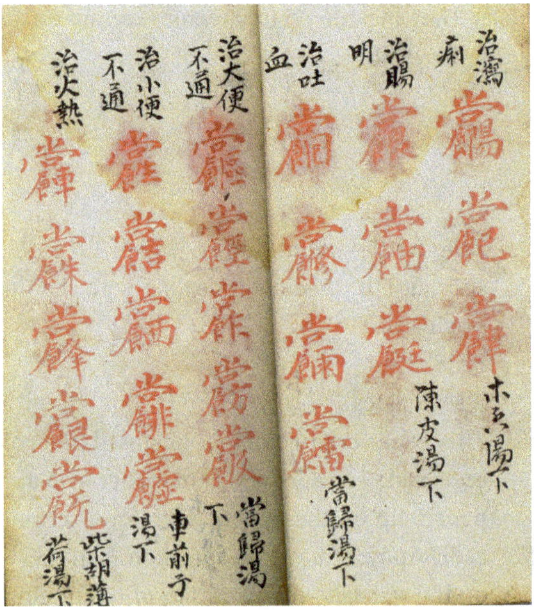

治濁　治痢　治賜明　治吐血

治大便不通　治小便不通　治火熱

陳皮湯下　　當歸湯下　　木瓜湯下

車前子　柴胡湯下　荷湯下

| TITLE PAGE: | With inscription: 增補祝由十三科. Back of title page, inscription: 軒轅碑記醫學祝由十三科/後附方便便方/京都琉璃廠善成堂發兌/西蜀青城山空青洞天藏版 |
| --- | --- |
| NO. OF PAGES: | 54 |
| L.P. /CH.L: | 6 x 19 |

LAYOUT:        No lines, no frames
AUTHOR AND YEAR OF TEXT:
        Unknown, Qing.
YEAR OF COPY:   Character 玄 written with final stroke omitted. Presumably Qing dynasty.

SURVEY OF CONTENTS: This volume is devoted to apotropaic therapy, referred to here as the medical "specialty of invocation of the origins", *zhu you ke* 祝由科. The title page states that the volume ends with an attachment of recipes, but this is not the case. As it refers to its source text as Jing du liu li chang shan cheng tang fa dui 京都琉璃廠善成堂發兌, "issued in the Capital by Shancheng tang in Liulichang", it is obvious that this is a copy of a printed book.

Historically, the "specialty of invocation of the origins" was an official specialty within regular Chinese medicine. Hence its texts were published in printed books and widely disseminated in society. The present volume is an example of such *zhu you ke* 祝由科 literature that is both very rich and complete in contents.

It begins with two paragraphs: 軒轅黃帝祝由科敍 and 軒轅黃帝祝由科序, signed with 涵谷山人體真子拜題. They are followed by a "List of 13 specialties within the specialty of invocation of the origins of Heavenly Physicians", Zhu you ke tian yi she san ke mu lu 祝由科天醫十三科目錄. The sub-branches distinguished here include: 大方脈、諸風科、胎產科、眼目科、小兒科、口齒科、痘疹科、傷折科、耳鼻科、瘡腫科、金鏃科、書禁科、砭鍼科.

The main text of the volume is preceded by "divine invocation texts for invocation of the origins", Zhu you shen zhou wen 祝由神咒文, including an "invocation to [prepare] the water [to dissolve ink to write an] invocation", *zhou shui zhou* 咒水咒; "invocation to [prepare] the ink [for writing an] invocation", *zhu mo zhou* 祝墨咒, "invocation to [prepare] the paper [for writing an] invocation", *zhu zhi zhou* 祝紙咒; "invocation to [prepare] the pen [for writing an] invocation", *zhu bi zhou* 祝筆咒; "invocation text", *zhu wen* 祝文, "invocation for writing a charm", *shu fu zhou* 書符咒; and "to send off the text", *song wen* 送文. These are steps to be followed in the course of preparing written charms.

This section is followed by 80 apotropaic recipes to cure disease. The therapeutic indication is written above the recipe. In the middle of the pages a "character charm" is drawn with red ink. Below this a pharmaceutical substance is recorded to be ingested as a decoction together with the charm. For most diseases numerous such "character charms" are to be written. In some instances one single "character charm" is suggested for use. The charms written on paper are to be burned to ashes and then to be swallowed with an acquaeous liquid or wine. Some of the recipes also include so-called "secret thunder instructions", *lei jue* 雷訣 and sword gestures.

The second half of the volume begins with a "sagely announcement by the true gentleman of noble grace", 崇恩真君聖誥. This is different from the preceding apotropaic contents. The announcement states 派流西地，跡顯龍興...修至道鐵師之教，掌玉府之雷書...光天南派五雷天心正法祝由科. The following text includes He qi zhi bing zhen fu jue fa 合氣治病真符訣法, "Patterns of secrect instructions on [the preparation of] genuine charms to cure disease by joining the Qi", with some "character charms", and also "graphic charms". The sequence of distinguishing between Yin and Yang ailments, voicing invocations, and writing charms greatly differs from the preceding "Thirteen specialties (or: 13th specialty) of Xian Yuan's invocation of the origins", Xian Yuan zhu you shi san ke 軒轅祝由十三科.。

The "character charms" advocated in this section are more complex than those in the first part. Also, an accompanying text explains the meaning of each character charm. The charms, as before, may be ingested together with a decoction of a pharmaceutical substance.

Following the "specialty of invocation of the origins as developed by the Bright Sky Southern School", *guang tian nan pai zhu you ke* 光天南派祝由科, a new section bears the title Tai ji zuo gong xian weng zhi wan bing fu jue 太極左宮仙翁治萬病符訣, "Secret instructions of the venerable hermit from the palace to the left of Tai Ji on charms to cure a myriad diseases". For this school the text states: 天臺得道，閫造成真。昔受東華，復傳西蜀, "Tian Yi obtained this Dao and transformed it for application in reality. Originally it was received in the East of China. It was then further transmitted to Shu in the West". Its therapeutic advice is offered in three sections, upper section *shang bu* 上部, central section *zhong bu* 中部, and lower section *xia bu* 下部. The use of charms for treating numerous diseases is part of all of them. The charms drawn here have some peculiarities. They are divided into *shang bu ling zhuan* 上部靈篆, "magic seals, upper section", *zhong bu ling zhuan* 中部靈篆, "magic seals, central section", and *xia bu ling zhuan* 下部靈篆, "magic seals, lower sections". The text also lists *wu xing wu dao wei zang yao* 五行五道為臟藥, "medication for the [body's] long-term depots based on the five phases and the five *dao*", as well as *sui zheng fu wei yao* 隨症符為藥, "amulets responding to individual signs of disease to be used as medication", in all with 96 charms. The therapies recorded are both simple and easy to understand.

Seen as a whole, this is a most encompassing and representative volume of *zhu you ke* 祝由科, "the specialty of invocation of the origins".

*** 

| | |
|---|---|
| TITLE: | *Hei shen wan* 黑神丸, Black spirit pill |
| ID: | 8939 |
| CONTENTS: | Gynecology |
| APPEARANCE: | Large size simple folk manuscript volume. Average calligraphy. Kraft paper cover added by later hand with new binding. No title. |
| BINDING: | Thread |
| MEASURE: | 25.3 x 21.2 |
| TITLE PAGE: | No |
| NO. OF PAGES: | 13 |
| L.P. /CH.L: | 11 x 21. Size of characters varies. |
| LAYOUT: | No lines, no borders |
| AUTHOR AND YEAR OF TEXT: | |
| | Wu Renhe 無任何. Year unknown. |

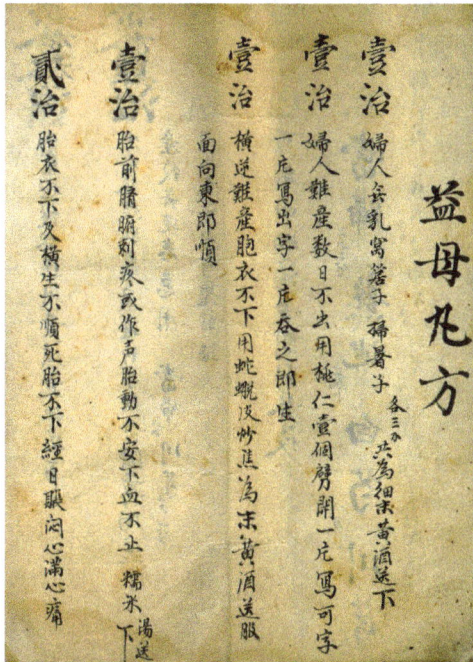

YEAR OF COPY:    Character 玄 not written to observe the Qing dynasty taboo. Republican era.

SURVEY OF CONTENTS: The first line of the text reads: 黑神丸專治臺前産後柒拾有餘証, "Black Spirit Pill to specifically cure more than 70 conditions before and after delivery". This is followed by a list of the components of this pill: *dang gui* 當歸, *mu xiang* 木香, *tian ma* 天麻, *jin mo* 金墨, *fei luo mian* 飛羅麵, *bai cao shuang* 百草霜. This then is followed by 74 "cures", *zhi* 治, i.e., 74 therapeutic indications and advice on the application of the Black Spirit Pill with modified ingredients. The volume concludes with a reference to a "recipe for a pill with *yi mu*", *yi mu wan fang* 益母丸方, and a list of 15 "cures". However, the ingredients of this recipe are not provided.

The Black Spirit Pills, and also the Black Gold Pills, received wide-spread attention during the Qing dynasty. The basic idea was always to have a key formula and adapt it, by adding or removing recipe components, to specific gynecological ailments.

***

TITLE:                (*Yao fang za chao* 藥方雜抄, Copy of miscellaneous pharmaceutical recipes)

ID:                   8940

CONTENTS:             Pharmaceutical recipes

APPEARANCE:           Poor, simple folk manuscript volume, without cover. No preface, no table of contents. Average calligraphy.

BINDING:              Paper spills

MEASURE:              21.4 x 114.4

TITLE PAGE:           No

NO. OF PAGES:         33

L.P. /CH.L:           Uneven. Mostly 9 x 20

LAYOUT:               No lines, no frames

AUTHOR AND YEAR OF TEXT:

                      Wu Renhe 無任何

YEAR OF COPY:         The text refers to recipes introduced by Wang Qingren 王清任 towards the end of the Qing dynasty. Republican era.

SURVEY OF CONTENTS: This volume is a folk record of miscellaneous recipes. Some of the therapeutic indications given for these recipes are worded in folk terms, such as *du teng* 肚疼, for "abdominal pain", and *nü ren ji zhua feng shou chou* 女人雞爪風手抽, "'Chicken claw wind' and 'hands pulled out' of women", referring to ailments that make a woman's fingers look fixed like a chicken claw, or stretched out straight and cramped. The recipes, though, are mostly those from regular Chinese medicine, including *xue fu zhu yu tang* 血府逐瘀湯, "decoction to expel stasis from the blood palace", *ge xia zhu yu tang* 隔下逐瘀湯, "decoction to expel stasis from below the diaphragm", etc. Other recipes are for ailments of the eyes, blood in the urine of a mule colt, abortion, preparation of bean curd, apotropaic purposes, and "to minimize the outbreak of pox", *xi dou* 稀痘. The disorderly structure and the miscellaneous contents of this volume suggest that it was prepared by a private person casually noting items that had come to his attention.

***

TITLE:            *Za lan. San shi liu she tai* 雜覽三十六舌胎, Various observa-
                  tions. Thirty six tongue coatings

ID:               8941

CONTENTS:         Tongue diagnosis

APPEARANCE:       Poor, simple manuscript. Average calligraphy. Cover made
                  from an old almanac page; severely torn. Two characters
                  faintly readable: 雜覽.

BINDING:          Thread

MEASURE:          21.2 x 14.5

TITLE PAGE:       No

NO. OF PAGES:     24

L.P. /CH.L:       Upper half of each page: tongue illustration; lower half 4 – 8
                  lines explanatory text. Latter half 9 x 20.

LAYOUT:           No lines, no frames

AUTHOR AND YEAR OF TEXT:

                  Unknown

YEAR OF COPY:     Character 玄 not written to observe the Qing dynasty taboo.
                  This, the quality of the paper, and the contents suggest that
                  this volume was written during the Republican era.

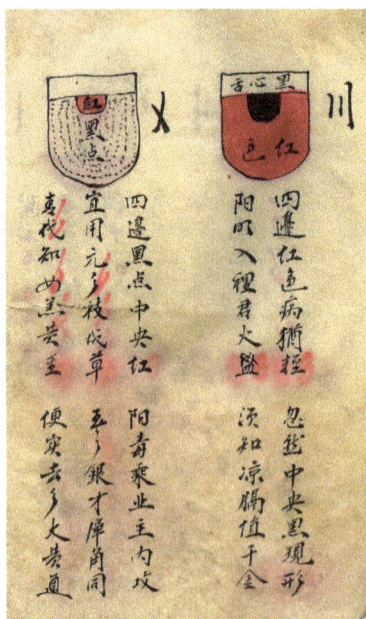

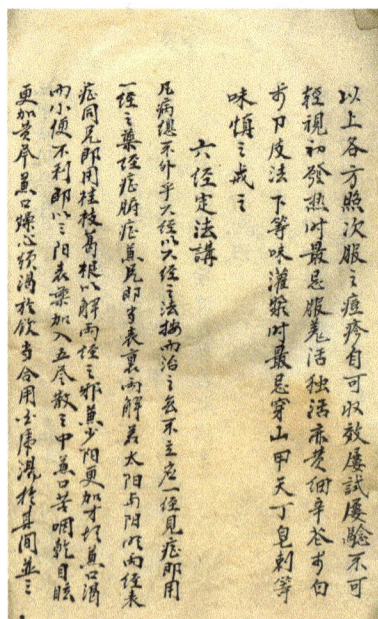

SURVEY OF CONTENTS: This manuscript volume has a first part on tongue diagnosis, and the second on diagnosis and therapy of miscellaneous illnesses.

The first section has 36 drawings of tongue conditions; the initial 14 drawings are colored with red ink; the remaining are black and white. Different sections of the tongue surface are identified with lines, and with written hints at their pathological coloring. The initial drawings show a tongue with a round tip. Later on the tongues are depicted as squares. Their sequence is numbered with the *hua ma* 花碼 numbering system. The explanatory text is rhymed; it explains the diaseases responsible for each tongue condition, and an appropriate pharmaceutical treatment.

The second part of the volume includes the following paragraphs: 五運、六氣、十二經瀉火藥、十二經虛實補瀉藥、治痘疹發論訣、催痘出齊方、千金內托散、六經定法講、通用湯方歌、聞聲、吐瀉不治歌、五指冷熱歌、四脈主病、總括脈要歌、脈證宜忌歌、卓溪家傳秘訣、入門審喉歌訣、藥王徑. Most of these paragraphs of rather heterogenous contents are written as rhymed verses.

Most conspicuous in this volume is the section on tongue diagnosis. The design of the drawings and their coloring are rarely encountered in such folk manuscripts.

***

| | |
|---|---|
| TITLE: | (*Dui lian. Yao fang za chao* 對聯、藥方雜抄. Couplets. Manuscript copy of miscellaneous recipes) |
| ID: | 8942 |
| CONTENTS: | Couplets, pharmaceutical recipes |
| APPEARANCE: | Ancient manuscript volume. Edges torn and bent. Deficient calligraphy. |
| BINDING: | Thread |
| MEASURE: | 24.5 x 13.4 |
| TITLE PAGE: | No |
| NO. OF PAGES: | 64 |
| L.P. /CH.L: | Uneven. Characters of different sizes. From 3-4 x >10, to 5-6 x approx.. 16 |
| LAYOUT: | No lines, no frames |

AUTHOR AND YEAR OF TEXT:

Unknown, last page with three naively cut personal seals: 歸太原.

YEAR OF COPY:   No Qing dynasty taboos observed. Contents dating from the end of the Qing dynasty. Republican era.

SURVEY OF CONTENTS: The first 32 pages list a large number of couplets as they are commonly used in businesses and private homes. There is also a pattern how to announce one's mother's death: 喪母引狀式. All this is unrelated to medicine.

Another 32 pages are devoted to medicine and pharmaceutical treatments, with tens of recipes. Therapeutic indications include 蝎子蜇人的符咒方、瘟疫、疥瘡、禿瘡、誤吃毒藥、婦人乾癆、無名腫毒、腹內生蟲、多年連瘡、咽喉、胃氣疼. There are charm and incantation recipes named 吃信方, "recipes for [treating the effects of] ingesting arsenic", 補心湯, "decoction to supplement the heart", 七厘散, "powder with seven minute amounts", 治吃洋煙, "to cure opium addiction", and 治犬咬傷方, "recipe to cure injuries resulting from dog bites". The recipes listed are of different types, and follow no standard norm or systematic sequence. They appear to have been recorded casually, as they came to the attention of the author of this volume. The volume thus is a common folk manuscript record.

\*\*\*

| | |
|---|---|
| TITLE: | *Za zheng* 杂症, Miscellaneous pathological conditions |
| ID: | 8943 |
| CONTENTS: | Pharmaceutical recipes |
| APPEARANCE: | Poor ancient manuscript volume with some damage. Text complete. Average calligraphy. Cover with inscription with two abbreviated characters: 杂症/信陽 |
| BINDING: | Thread |
| MEASURE: | 21 x 14.1 |
| TITLE PAGE: | No |
| NO. OF PAGES: | 23 |
| L.P. /CH.L: | Uneven. Approx. 8 x 24 |
| LAYOUT: | No lines, no frames |
| AUTHOR AND YEAR OF TEXT: | |
| | Unknown |

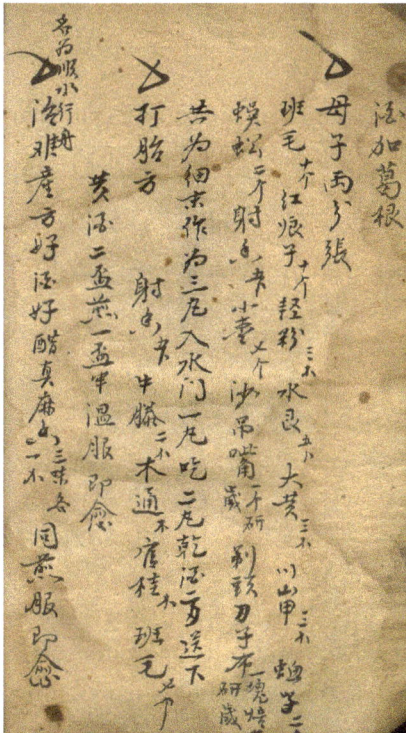

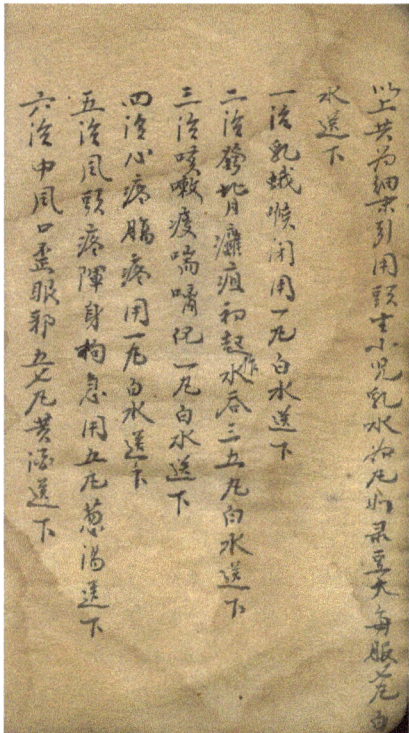

YEAR OF COPY:    Character 痰 written to observe a Qing dynasty taboo. Other relevant characters not written to observe Qing dynasty taboos. This and the paper quality suggest that this volume was written in the Republican era.

SURVEY OF CONTENTS: This volume at its beginning has a table of contents showing that this is a collection of 63 pharmaceutical recipes. The therapeutic indications mostly are those from the realms of external medicine and gynecology. They include both regular fixed recipes and folk single ingredient recipes. The pharmaceutical substances required are mostly those sold in pharmaceutical shops. Others are items of daily use, such as ox horns, a male dog's head, chicken, and geese. Recipes for abortion have names such as *mu zi liang fen zhang* 母子兩分張, and *da tai fang* 打胎方. Following the 63 recipes of the main text a further list of more than ten recipes was recorded by a different hand.

***

TITLE:    *Wen yi he bian* 瘟疫合编, A summary on warmth epidemics
ID:    8944
CONTENTS:    Warmth disease
APPEARANCE:    Ancient manuscript volume. Calligraphy deficient. Cover made of common paper, with inscription: 瘟疫合編下函/緒生堂段記.
BINDING:    Thread
MEASURE:    17.4 x 11.5
TITLE PAGE:    Inscription: 增補傷寒瘟疫合辨卷四五六.
NO. OF PAGES:    67
L.P. /CH.L:    8 x approx. 23
LAYOUT:    No lines, no frames
AUTHOR AND YEAR OF TEXT:
    Yang Xuan 杨璿 (Lishan 栗山, Yuheng 玉衡); Qing dynasty.
YEAR OF COPY:    Republican era. Character 玄 not written to observe the Qing dynasty taboo. But continuation of drug names introduced to obey the taboo, such as *yuan shen* 元參.

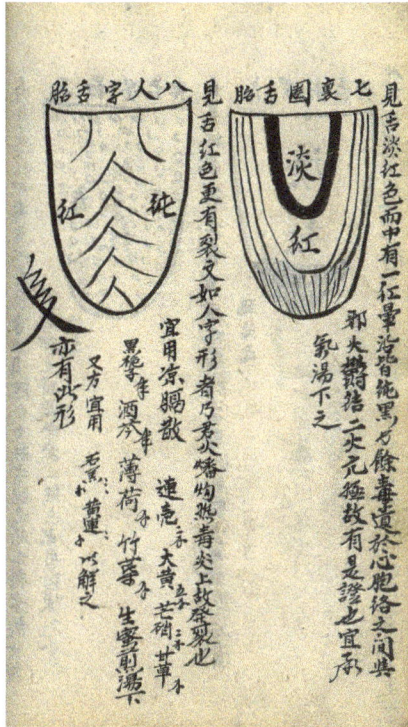

SURVEY OF CONTENTS: This volume is a fragmentary copy of *juan* 4, 5, and 6 of possibly the Qing author Yang Xuan's 杨璿 *Shang han wen yi tiao bian* 傷寒瘟疫條辨. Apparently, the copyist added further contents. All of this remains to be researched. The volume has neither a table of contents nor a preface or an afterword. It begins with more than 10 paragraphs on warmth epidemics; the initial ones having the titles: 補陰症、補陽症、三復、發腫. This is followed by a heading 瘟疫明辨後序方目錄四, listing 84 recipes with therapeutic indication and each formula's components.

Next are 36 black and white drawings of tongue conditions, with different colors indicated by the respective words. To the side of the drawings the author added an explanatory text, as well as therapeutic advice on how to treat the underlying disease. This section is followed again by a list of more than ten pharmaceutical recipes, including those for treating oxes and horses with warmth disease.

This volume was written by the same hand as ms. 8953.

***

TITLE:            *Zhi yan quan ke* 治眼全科, complete ophthalmological specialty

ID:               8945

CONTENTS:         Ophthalmology

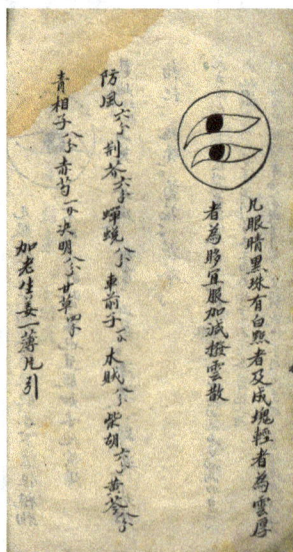

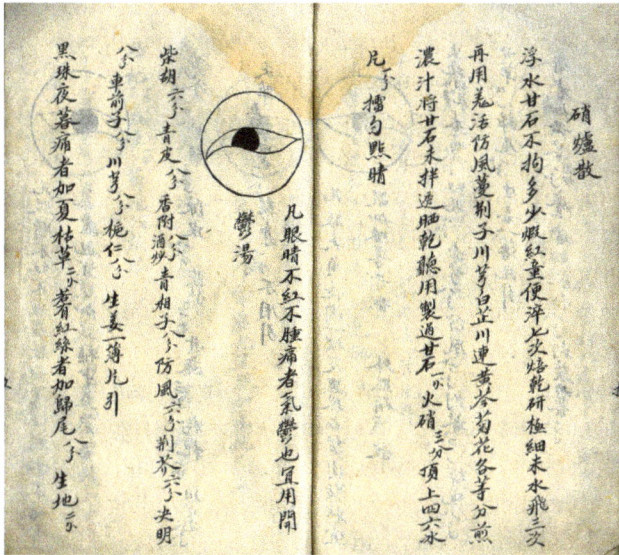

APPEARANCE: Relatively well preserved manuscript volume with exceptional calligraphy. Cover paper prepared from kapok, with inscription: 治眼全科壹部/玉選記. Inside of front cover, inscription: 六月十八日立.

BINDING: Thread

MEASURE: 22.4 x 13.2

TITLE PAGE: No

NO. OF PAGES: 16

L.P. /CH.L: 5 – 7 x approx. 23

LAYOUT: No lines, no frames

AUTHOR AND YEAR OF TEXT:

Cheng Songya 程松崖, ca. 1484. Personal name of copyist: Yuxuan 玉選. Family name unknown.

YEAR OF COPY: This volume is a manuscript copy of a printed book printed in the *guang xu* 光緒 reign period, *xin si* 辛巳 year, i.e., 1881. The character 絃 is not written to observe the Qing dynasty taboo. Republican era.

SURVEY OF CONTENTS: This volume has a preface written in the 13th year of the *tong zhi* 同治 reign period by a man with a self-given style name Shouzhuosheng 守拙生, "the lad who preserves his ignorance", identified as a lower official, *shi zhi* 使署, at a place called San yuan 三原. From this preface one learns that the present manuscript volume's printed source text is the Ming author Cheng Songya's 程松崖 *Yan ke ying yan liang fang* 眼科应验良方. A second preface is introduced by the following lines: 光緒辛巳......古滇味道縣省新氏書于愛雪堂, "During the *guang xu* reign period, in the *xin si* year (i.e., 1881), ...written by Mr. Competence-in-what-is-new, from Wei dao county in old Yunnan". A line following this preface states: 程松崖先生眼科应验良方敘, "preface of Mr. Cheng Songya's Proven and Good Recipes in Ophthalmology", but this preface was not copied.

The main text begins with a drawing of the human eye, identifying its associations with the five organs heart, lung, liver, kidneys and spleen, as well as the stomach. This is followed by another 17 drawings, 13 of which show no pathological changes. Only the final 4 drawings are designed to depict the appearance of disease. These drawings are then accompanied by text explaining the ailments, and their pharmaceutical therapy, including the components of the recipes recommended for treatment.

*** 

| | |
|---|---|
| TITLE: | *Tu zhu yan ke* 图注眼科, Illustrated ophthalmology |
| ID: | 8946 |
| CONTENTS: | Ophthalmology |
| APPEARANCE: | Ancient manuscript volume. New cover of kraft paper pasted around the back. Inscription on cover with abbreviated characters: 图注眼科/手抄. |
| BINDING: | Paper spills |
| MEASURE: | 23.5 x 13.3 |
| TITLE PAGE: | No |
| NO. OF PAGES: | 16 |
| L.P. /CH.L: | Uneven. Average: 4-7 x 15-18 |
| LAYOUT: | No lines, no frames |
| AUTHOR AND YEAR OF TEXT: | |
| | Cheng Songya 程松崖, ca. 1484. |
| YEAR OF COPY: | Republican era. Character 弦 not written to observe the Qing dynasty taboo. |

SURVEY OF CONTENTS: The first line of the main text states: *Yan ke ge fang* 眼科各方, "all recipes in ophthalmology". This is followed by a drawing of the human eye with characters in the drawing and a text underneath identifying

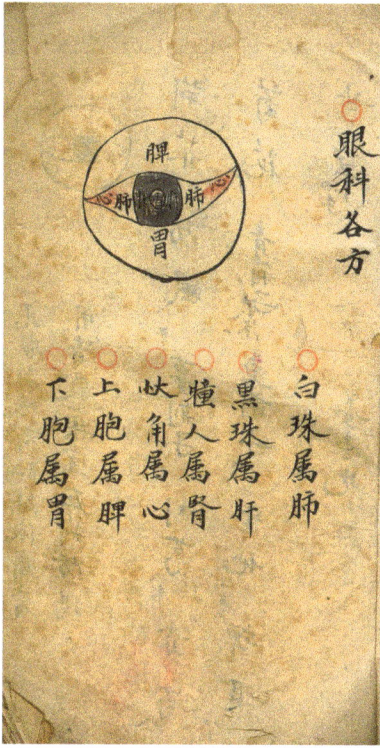

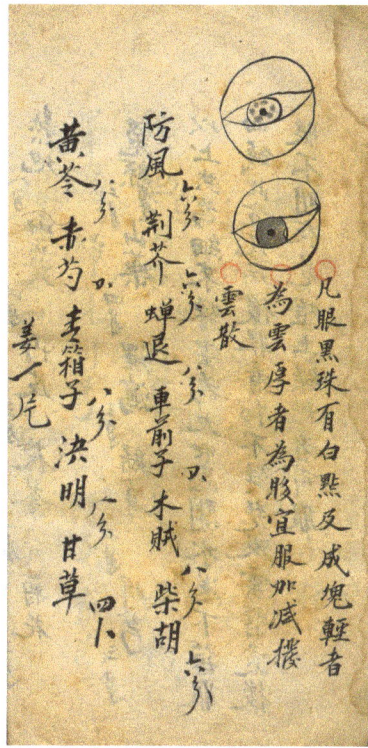

correspondences between the sections of the eye and internal organs. This is followed by another 17 drawings, some of them showing pathological changes marked with red ink, such as red vessels permeating the eye, or normally white sections now turned red. From the text it is obvious that this is a copy of the Ming author Cheng Songya's 程松崖 *Yan ke jing yan liang fang* 眼科应验良方. However, the copyist did not follow his source book in the sequence of the ailments recorded.

***

| | |
|---|---|
| TITLE: | (*Yao fang chao ben* 藥方抄本, Manuscript volume of pharmaceutical recipes) |
| ID: | 8947 |
| CONTENTS: | Pharmaceutical recipes; apotropaics |
| APPEARANCE: | Ancient manuscript volume. Average calligraphy. Cover made from locally produced paper, mulberry paper. No in- |

scription. One seal, square, characters illegible. Edges worn.
Text complete.

| | |
|---|---|
| BINDING: | Thread |
| MEASURE: | 21.2 x 14.0 |
| TITLE PAGE: | No |
| NO. OF PAGES: | 53 |
| L.P. /CH.L: | 8 x approx. 18 |
| LAYOUT: | Red column lines and frame 17.2 x 12.5, |

AUTHOR AND YEAR OF TEXT:

Unknown

YEAR OF COPY: End of Qing dynasty/early Republican era. Character 痰 written to obey Qing dynasty taboo. The text includes several recipes that were introduced towards the end of the Qing dynasty. Although a writing during the Qing era is possible, the use of paper with red column lines and frame suggests a more recent date.

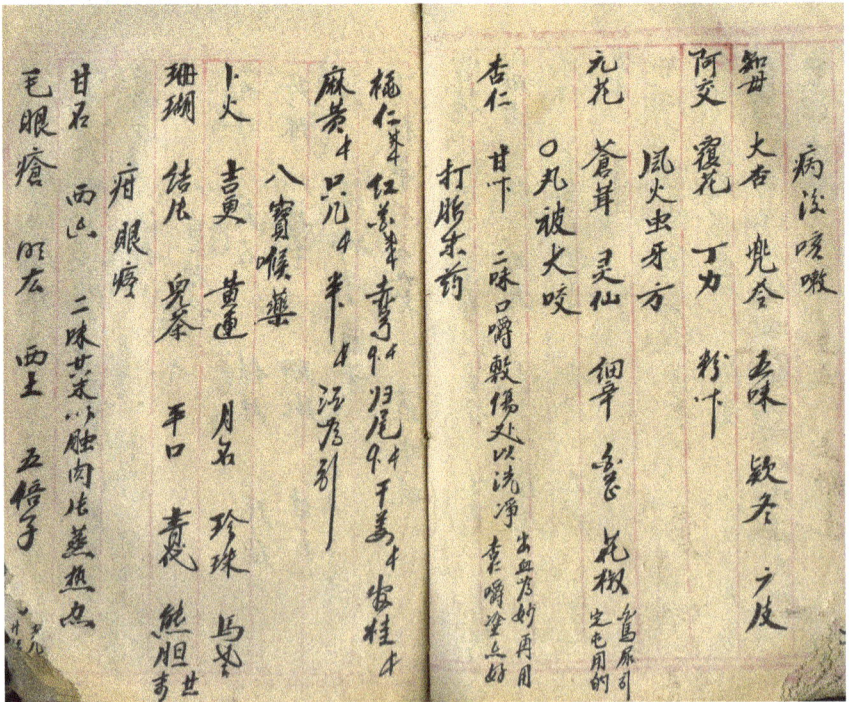

SURVEY OF CONTENTS: The entire volume is devoted to pharmaceutical and apotropaic recipes. The sequence of the recipes follows no categorization of therapeutic indications. However, a general structure is recognizable. The text begins with tens of fixed pharmaceutical recipes, such as *liu wei di huang wan* 六味地黃丸, and *ba wei di huang wan* 八味地黃丸. They are followed by again tens of decoction recipes. These in turn are followed by apotropaic formulae, recipes for injuries received through blows and falls, further recipes from external medicine, recipes for various pathological conditions, as well as those from the realms of gynecology and pediatrics. In all, the volume records more than 200 recipes.

The apotropaic recipes are mostly those of the "character charms" type. They do not include any oral spells. Their therapeutic indications include: *ru teng* 乳疼, "breast pain", *zhi xue* 止血, "to stop bleeding", *zhi teng* 止疼, "to stop pain", *jie gu* 接骨, "bone-setting", *cui sheng* 催生, "to hasten delivery", *she yao* 蛇咬, "snake bite"; *ya chi teng* 牙齒疼, "toothache", *feng gou yao* 瘋狗咬, "rabies dog's bite", *yin jian* 陰箭, "invisible arrow" (a folk term for sudden muscular pain).

Among the pharmaceutical recipes one finds advice for abortion, as is frequently documented in folk manuscripts. Examples from the current volume are *zhuan da tai ling yan fang* 專打胎靈驗方, "magically effective recipe for specifically smashing the fetus", and *da tai mo yao* 打胎末藥, "powder medication for smashing the fetus".

The names of pharmaceutical drugs are often not those used in regular Chinese pharmacy. The copyist used abbreviated names instead, as they are commonly found in folk manuscripts. Examples are *jie geng* 吉更 for 桔梗; *chuan xia* 川下 for *chuan xia* 川夏; *qian shi* 芡十 for *qian shi* 芡實; *xiang fu* 香付 for 香附; *ren shan* 人乡 for *ren shen* 人參; *yuan zhao* 元召 for *lian qiao* 連翹; *hu bo* 虎白 for 琥珀; *qing dai* 青代 for 青黛; *ba mao* 八毛 for *ban mao* 斑蝥; *hong liang* 紅良 for *hong niang zi* 紅娘子; *a wei* 阿味 for 阿魏, and *zhai nan* 宅南 for *ze lan* 澤蘭.

The names of diseases are mostly those found in books of regular Chinese medicine. However, the text also includes secret names used by the people. An example is *ma ma teng* 媽媽疼, lit.: "mama pain". From the recipe recommended this should be abscesses of the female breast.

Among the recipes is one *wu tun yan tu fang* 誤吞煙土方, "recipe for having inadvertently ingested opium", and the *Lin Wenchong gong jie yang yan fang* 林文忠公戒洋煙方, "Sir Lin Wenchong's recipe to give up opium". This is evidence that the present volume must have been written after the Opium Wars.

***

| | |
|---|---|
| TITLE: | (*Fang shu chao* 方書抄; Manuscript copy of recipe literature) |
| ID: | 8948 |
| CONTENTS: | Pharmaceutical recipes |
| APPEARANCE: | Large size manuscript volume. Original cover lost. New cover made of kraft paper thread-bound to the original manuscript. Edges severely torn. Text complete. Cover without inscription. Main text written by numerous hands. Calligraphy at times average, at times deficient. First page with three seals: One of ellipse form with three characters cut in relief: 端居室. Another in oval form, also with characters cut in relief: 河間長垣劉茁字伯行. The third shows a human figure, cut in intaglio, its characters illegible. |
| BINDING: | Thread |
| MEASURE: | 23.6 x 27.0 |
| TITLE PAGE: | No |
| NO. OF PAGES: | 26 |
| L.P. /CH.L: | 16 x approx. 20 |
| LAYOUT: | No lines, no frames |
| AUTHOR AND YEAR OF TEXT: | |
| | Unknown |
| YEAR OF COPY: | Republican era. Character 玄 not written to obey the Qing dynasty taboo. |

SURVEY OF CONTENTS: The first half of this volume is a list of pharmaceutical recipes that appear to have been copied from a printed medical book. Hence the recipes follow a categorization along groups of therapeutic indications. Their sequence is as follows : "Department of divinely effective external specialty", *shen xiao wai ke men* 神效外科門 (91 recipes); "Department of 100 pediatric ailments", *xiao er bai bing men* 小兒百病門 (15 recipes); "Department of eyes, mouth, and teeth", *yan mu kou chi men* 眼目口齒門 (15 recipes, plus 14 miscellaneous recipes); "Department of filling depletion and taking care of injuries", *bu yi xu sun men* 補益虛損門 (8 recipes) plus 59 others.

The second half of this volume is introduced by the heading: Yi fang ze yao wai ke za zheng 醫方擇要外科雜症, "A choice of important medical recipes for miscellaneous illness conditions in external medicine", followed by a list of 52 recipes for miscellaneous therapeutic indications.

Most of the recipes recorded are fixed recipes copied from printed books. Some are recipes solely transmitted among the common people. This includes, for example, aphrodisiacs that would never have found entrance into printed books. This also includes typical folk recipes with one single component not found in regular materia medica. An example is a *lian chuang fang* 臁瘡方, "recipe for shank sores". It uses "pieces scooped by a veterinarian from the hoof of a donkey. They are to be roasted in an earthenware pot, maintaining their nature, and ground to powder. If [the sores are] moist, [the powder] is to be applied dried. If [the sores are] dry, it is to be mixed with *ma you* and then applied."

紫黑疔瘡起内是有空蛇頭疔生于指尖疼痛
多骨瘡内有格大截頸瘡似有横列刀形相
入而瘡王化膝而益紅腫高大氣色亦足有口吃
久積陰瘡有管眼者必
形即爛時馬道瘡生于鼻内久則孔内有膿
刮臭爛瘡生于口喉用塵舌耀明齒内有泡点紅
魚鱗瘡爛咳嗽吐膿水為輕症
走馬牙疳生于上牙唇腮不疼微有黑腮
紅口瘡流痧水為
白口瘡齒熱無痧水為
喉白一粒珠
喉驚為單鎖喉

雙鵝為閉鎖唯如不能重舌舌底似長一小吉
奶癖七藏以内為奶癖次指有線
藏癖心藏以外為藏癖男子生左肋下女生右
氣癧肋下堅硬形如栗子摊之無根不破日久俗名左鼠瘡日流膿
瘰癧即氣瘕破者為癙瘡日流膿
痔瘡生腹内左為瘊右為痕
魚口生小肚子旁居左便毒生小肚旁居右便
楊梅瘡内有泡照花桂頂白根赤用指重捻手心便是凝結者凡

○瘟病取穴先以紅布七層安穴上將針向火
燒透對正穴道安於布上俟藥氣漸透肌膝再
入病與便覺清爽效甚速若太熱將針提起俟
熱乏再針以七記數重則一至九多則六亦可針後
靜卧片時使藥氣周身暢達再量飲醇酒以行藥
氣切忌當風慎起居節飲食凡事調攝做以初
恣情縱欲以致不救于針無若人神在日不宜針
灸惟急症從權針後餘藥以乾竹筒收藏復用
審病取穴開列於左
百會穴 治中風頭風癲癇用弓反張健忘脱肛目瘈耳聾

上星穴 治臭瘤臭塞腦漏頭痛目疾多灸亦恐拔氣墮目
神庭穴 治目眩出淚泣風癇目腫目眩
天突穴 治喉瘡喉風哮喘氣噎肺癰咯血喉中有聲
上脘穴 治心腹疼驚悸痰癖伏梁氣蠱奔豚風癇熱癖
中脘穴 治脾胃食脹滿如伏梁傷寒飲水過多腹脹氣喘
氣海穴 治陽癖臍下冷痛一切氣症
關元穴 治諸帶吐食脹滿氣或塊陰症痼冷水腫心腹脹脹疼
中極穴 治遺精白濁臍下冷痛小便頻數婦人帶經不調
臨泣穴 治目痛搶心遺泄失精五淋久卒小便赤澁經不調不受孕
客主穴 治頷頬痛内瘴亦目至眼邪手閉牽閉失音不語

***

TITLE:        (*Wai ke zhu bing zhi fang* 外科諸病治方, Recipes to treat all
              sorts of diseases in the realm of external medicine)

ID:                8949
CONTENTS:          External medicine
APPEARANCE:        Thin, poor ancient manuscript volume. Edges on lower left severely damaged but text complete. Cover darkened by age. No inscription. Text: careful handwriting.
BINDING:           Paper spills
MEASURE:           18.4 x 13.0
TITLE PAGE:        No
NO. OF PAGES:      21
L.P. /CH.L:        10 x 20
LAYOUT:            No lines, no frames
AUTHOR AND YEAR OF TEXT:
                   Unknown
YEAR OF COPY:      Presumably late Qing. Character 玄 written to observe the Qing dynasty taboo.

SURVEY OF CONTENTS: The contents of this volume are quite mixed. It begins with a paragraph on obstruction-illness, *yong* 癰, ulcers, *yang* 瘍, and sores poison, *chuang du* 瘡毒, with the title Yin yang biao li lun 陰陽表裡論, "on Yin-, Yang-, outer and inner sections". Next is a section Kan fa lun 看法論, "on patterns of observing/diagnosing", listing conditions from external medicine such as *ju* 疽, impediment illness, *yong* 癰, obstruction illness, *ding* 疔, pin-illness; *chuang* 瘡, sores; *pi* 癖, aggregation-illness, *luo li* 瘰癧, scrofula; *pi ji* 痞積, obstacle-illness accumulation; and *liu* 瘤, tumor, with simple descriptions of their appearance. This is followed by a section Zhi fa lun 治法論, "on patterns of treating", with a discourse on the treatment of sores and abscesses in external medicine. Next are lists of 32 frequently used recipes for sores and abscesses in external medicine, such as the *nei tuo tang* 內托湯, "decoction to uphold internally", the *ba zhen tang* 八珍湯, "decoction with eight juwels", and two recipes in an appendix.

These paragraphs are succeeded by the following paragraphs: 太乙神針, "Tai yi's divine needle" (referring to moxibustion sticks), 審病取穴, "Examine the disease and select [appropriate] insertion holes" (with a listing of 31 insertion points for symptom-guided acupuncture), 逐日人神所在不宜針灸, "A list of locations, changing daily, where the spirit resides and where it is not appropriate to needle or cauterize", 熨癖積瘰癧方, "recipes of compresses to treat aggregation-illness accumulation and scrofula", 熨純陰瘡方, "recipes for pure yin sores", 熨純陽瘡方, "recipes for pure yang sores", 熨大麻風方, „recipes for hot compresses to be applied in the treatment of Great Numbing Wind (i.e., leprosy)".

Seen as a whole, this book focusses on therapy patterns (pharmaceutical recipes, moxibustion, acupuncture, hot compresses) applied in external medicine. The handwriting is careful but writing errors are very many. Perhaps this volume was written by a person with a rather high level of formal education but who was an amateur in the field of external medicine nevertheless.

***

TITLE:                  *Ma ke yi jie* 麻科易解, Easy explanations from the [therapeutic] specialty concerned with measles, with an appendix: *Er ke za zhi* 兒科雜治, Pediatrics: miscellaneous cures
ID:                     8950
CONTENTS:               Pediatrics
APPEARANCE:             Very nice example of an ancient manuscript volume. Exceptionally beautiful calligraphy of formal script written in very small characters. Cover: tough paper made from the bast of paper mulberry. Inscription with brush: 麻科易解附兒科雜治，玖樽氏手錄（全）/玖樽氏. Two rectangular, red seals, characters carved in relief. The first: 治古同囚？固圖書珍藏. Below this one the second: 陳久尊章.
BINDING:                Originally paper spills; later added thread.
MEASURE:                19.2 x 12.9
TITLE PAGE:             No
NO. OF PAGES:           *Ma ke yi jie*: 13; *Er ke za zhi*: 12.
L.P. /CH.L:             12 x 24
LAYOUT:                 No lines, no frames
AUTHOR AND YEAR OF TEXT:
                        Liu Guishu 刘桂蔬, 1924. Copy by Mr. Jiu Zun 玖樽氏, (Chen Jiuzun 陳久尊).
YEAR OF COPY:           Republican era.

SURVEY OF CONTENTS: This is a manuscript copy of a printed book. However, the original author is not named. A comparision with the *Zhong guo zhong yi gu ji zong mu* 中國中醫古籍總目 shows that the source text was written by Liu Guishu 刘桂蔬 who published it in letterpress in 1924. The book was reprinted

麻子熱毒上攻咽喉不宜用針去刺有表邪閉住毒氣不散

蘇葉喉痛已經出了仍舊咳嗽是肺家有火用「清金率肺湯」加杏仁

還要咳嗽繼繼好不可固咳嗽設法止住祇是咳嗽太甚也不

相宜繼起的時候是風邪閉了用「宣毒發表湯」加杏仁

麻子多「咳嗽」毒邪可以借他散去所以麻子十日以內

或已經收了用「黃連解毒湯」

「喘急」是麻證最不好的氣象是表實毒氣閉在裏面不能夠出來用「清氣化毒飲」

出了這是毒氣內攻用「麻杏甘石湯」已經咳嗽

藥方

宣毒發表湯

葛根

牛蒡 各一錢

前胡

本通八分

蘇荷

竹葉 甘艸 各五分

枳壳

荊芥 北風

連翹 各一分

夏月不可加

裏熱加黃苓

寒邪加麻黃

古方有升麻桔梗這兩味藥都是上升的性怕他把邪勢

總宜禁用為是

部位 腦后 顖 太陽 頰 腮 臍 膝

later in Changsha 長沙 twice. Perhaps the author was based in that region. The copyist was extremely careful. Apparently he copied the entire text.

The *Ma ke yi jie* 麻科易解 is not divided into *juan* 卷. It is written in vernacular language und with modern chapters and sections, as well as punctuation. The major chapter headings are: 麻子的名稱, 麻子的傳染, 出麻的時候, 看護麻子與麻子的禁忌, 診麻子的總決, 驗出麻子的法子, etc. The text concludes with a list of 35 pharmaceutical recipes.

The *Er ke za zhi* mentioned on the cover has the full title: *Fu kan xiao er ke wai zhi ji ji man feng za zhi* 附刊小兒科外治及急慢驚風雜治. This part has a table of contents. These contents, though, are rather heterogenous, covering the following issues: Zhi fa 治法, "therapeutic methods", Fu you bian fan li 福幼編凡例, "introduction to the *Fu you bian*", 急慢驚風各種治法及藥方, "all sorts of therapeutic methods and pharmaceutical recipes for acute and chronic fright wind", You er kai kou fa 幼兒開口法, "a method to open the mouth of newborns" (i.e., having a newborn ingest medication to stimulate its discharge of waste remaining in its body from its time in the uterus), Ti tai tou fa 剃胎頭法, "a method to shave the hair of a newborn for the first time", Shi kou su fa 拭口穢法, "a method to wipe the dirt out of a newborn's mouth", and Xi dou fa 稀痘法, "a method to minimize the outbreak of smallpox". Such ideas and practices for prevention and therapy were widespread among the common people at the time.

***

TITLE:            *Yao shu* 藥書, Book on medication.
ID:               8951
CONTENTS:         Pharmaceutical recipes; apotropaics
APPEARANCE:       Ancient manuscript volume using paper with violet lines and frames. Average calligraphy. Cover made of dark paper with traces of burning heat. A loose recipe was glued to the inside of the back cover. Back cover with inscription in abbreviated characters: 药书, written by later owner.
BINDING:          Thread
MEASURE:          20.4 x 14.4
TITLE PAGE:       No
NO. OF PAGES:     45
L.P. /CH.L:       Approx. 6-8 x 20.
LAYOUT:           Paper with lines and frame, but not observed by writer.
AUTHOR AND YEAR OF TEXT:
                  Unknown
YEAR OF COPY:     Late Qing to early Republican era. In the early parts of the text, the character 玄 is written to observe the Qing dynasty taboo. In later sections there are occasional entries written with a fountain pen.

SURVEY OF CONTENTS: The first half of this volume is a record of pharmaceutical recipes. It has no table of contents, and the recipes are not categorized according to therapeutic indications. However, most of the recipes, these are the initial 47 entries, are advised for women's diseases. Several recipes are introduced by a description of their common therapeutic indications. Following the gynecological recipes a second section, *za zheng* 雜症, "miscellaneous conditions" comprises about 50 entries. The handwriting of these entries suggests that they were not recorded at one time or by one person only. One line states: 光緒十三年六月後，河南、陝州一帶白纏喉瘟疫大發，陶大尹刻方以救, "Beginning with the 6th month of the 13th year of the *guang xu* reign period in the

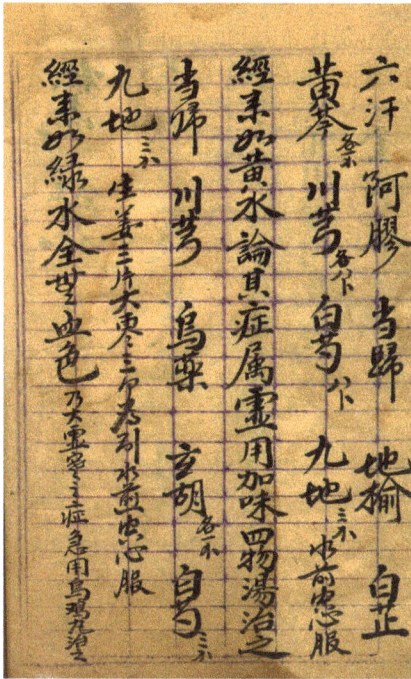

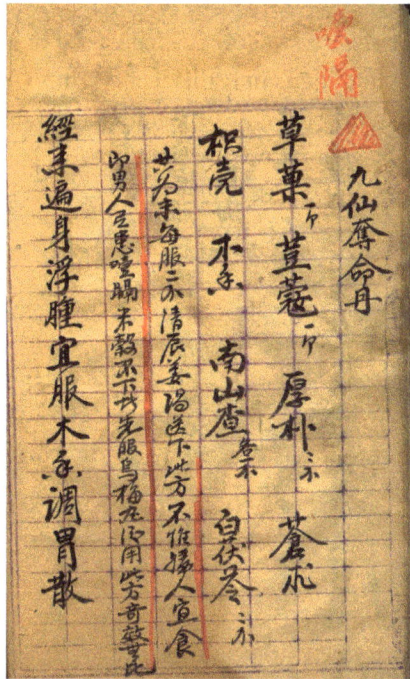

region of Henan, Shanzhou, a warmth epidemic of diphtheria broke out. Chief administrator Tao had this recipe carved to offer relief."

The pharmaceutical recipes are succeeded by apotropaic recipes. The therapeutic indications listed here include: *tie da sun shang* 跌打損傷, "injuries from blows and falls"; *chuang zhong* 瘡腫, "sores and swelling"; *huo luan tu xie* 霍亂吐瀉, "cholera with vomiting and outflow"; *xie zhe* 蝎蜇, "scorpion sting"; *chai nai* 吹奶, "breast inflation"; *nüe ji* 瘧疾, "malaria", *cui sheng* 催生, "to hasten delivery". The approach advocated is mostly an oral spell. Only two character charms and one graphic charm are recorded. Some of the oral spells are rather distinct and would not appear in printed books.

In the entry *jiu xian tuo ming dan* 九仙奪命丹, "Elixir of the Nine Immortals to snatch life", recommended to treat *ye ge* 噎嗝, esophagus cancer, the copyist used red ink to emphasize its importance. The entire entry reads: "*cao guo* 草果一個, *tsao guo* fruit, 1 specimen; *dou kou* 豆蔻, round cardamom, 1 specimen; *hou pu* 厚朴, magnolia bark, 3 qian; *cang zhu* 蒼朮, rhizome of atractylodes; *zhi qiao* 枳殼, citron/orange fruit; *mu xiang* 木香, saussurea root; *nan shan zha* 南山查, Southern crataegus fruit, 1 qian each; *bai fu ling* 白茯苓, white poria fungi, 2 qian. Together to be ground to powder. Each dosage 2 qian. To be ingested with ginger decoction in the early morning. This recipe is recommended to be taken not only by women. Males suffering from esophagus cancer and being unable to swallow rice/cereals should first ingest the 'pills with *wu mei*' 烏梅丸 and then apply this recipe. The extraordinary effects are incomparable." Apparently, the copyist regarded this recipe as most effective; an opinion possibly based on his own experience.

***

| | |
|---|---|
| TITLE: | *Dou chuang quan shu* 痘瘡全書, Complete text on pox sores |
| ID: | 8952 |
| CONTENTS: | Smallpox |
| APPEARANCE: | Ancient manuscript volume. Cover added by later hand. Inscription: 痘瘡全書. Paper of main text darkened by age. Small characters. Average calligraphy. Color or ink fading. |
| BINDING: | Thread |
| MEASURE: | 23.2 x 12.2 |
| TITLE PAGE: | No |
| NO. OF PAGES: | 78 |
| L.P. /CH.L: | 8 x 36 |
| LAYOUT: | No lines, no frames |
| AUTHOR AND YEAR OF TEXT: | |
| | Huang Lian 黃廉?, Ming dynasty |
| YEAR OF COPY: | Republican era. Character 玄 not written to observe the Qing dynasty taboo. |

SURVEY OF CONTENTS: This is a complete book on smallpox with 11 *juan*. It is possible though that additional sections are missing from this volume. No author and title are given for the main text. Hence the source text, presumably a printed book, is yet to be identified.

The very beginning may be lost. The text begins with 5 double pages 該卷先羅列西江月數十首 discussing therapy patterns for smallpox. Two further paragraphs on one double page appear to have been erroneously inserted here: Huang er bing 黃耳病 and Chi ge xiong 赤膈胸. They are not related to smallpox. Next is a section with the heading *juan* 1; it begins with three long sections: Yuan zhen fu 原疹賦, Dou chuang yuan liu 痘瘡源流, and Dou chuang zhi fa 痘瘡治法, followed by a more "general outline of the therapy of smallpox", Zhi dou zong kuo 治痘總括.

The sequence of the subsequent sections is as follows:

*Juan* 3: 發熱証治括; *juan* 4: 見形証治括; *juan* 5: 起發証治括; *juan* 6: 養漿成實証治括; *juan* 7: 收靨証治括; *juan* 8: 餘毒証治括; *juan* 9: 治疹西江月十三首; juan 10: 原疹論; juan11: 疹証治括.

An examination of the contents shows obvious similarities to the Ming author Huang Lian's 黃廉 *Dou zhen quan shu* 痘疹全書. However, beginning with *juan* 9, the issues dealt with are differentiated in even more detail. Hence the true source remains to be identified through a comparison with other such texts.

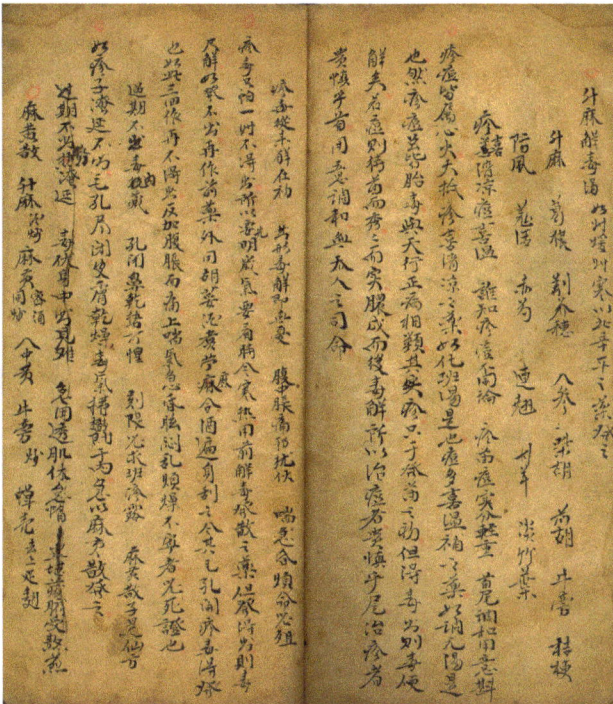

\*\*\*

| TITLE: | *Shang han she jian* 傷寒舌鑑, Harm caused by cold: the tongue is the mirror |
|---|---|
| ID: | 8953 |
| CONTENTS: | Tongue diagnosis |
| APPEARANCE: | Ancient manuscript volume. Careful handwriting. Good calligraphy. Cover with inscription: 傷寒舌鑑. |
| BINDING: | Thread |
| MEASURE: | 17.1 x 10.3 |

TITLE PAGE: No

NO. OF PAGES: Main text: 40. Recipes: 3

L.P. /CH.L: Uneven. Characters at times large, at times small. Approx. 8-14 x >24.

LAYOUT: No lines, no frames

AUTHOR AND YEAR OF TEXT:

Zhang Deng 張登, 1668. Copyist signed with Xu sheng tang 續生堂, Duan ji 段記, "apothecary to prolong life. Signed Duan".

YEAR OF COPY: Republican era. The copyist of this volume is identical with the copyist of another manuscript volume: *Wen yi he bian* 瘟疫合編, # 8944.

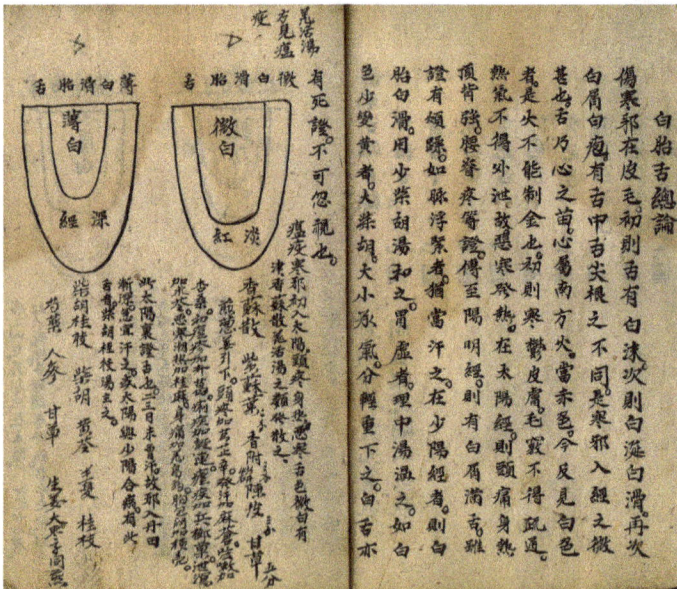

SURVEY OF CONTENTS: This is a complete copy of the Qing dynasty author Zhang Deng's 張登 *Shang han she jian* 傷寒舌鑒. Hence it begins with the author's "own preface", Zi xu 自序, signed 康熙戊申……張登. This is followed by a table of contents, signed again with the name Zhang Deng 張登. It lists nine categories of different tongue coatings, each with a specified number of sub-conditions: 白胎舌 (29); 黃胎舌 (17); 黑胎舌 (14); 灰色舌 (11); 紅色舌 (26); 紫色舌 (12); 黴醬色舌 (3); 藍色胎紋舌 (2); 妊娠傷寒舌 (6). Together these are 120 different pathological conditions. Each of them is shown on the subsequent pages with a black-and-white drawing in the upper half of each page indicating, often in great detail, the respective appearance of the tongue coating. Detailed descriptions, including advice on pharmaceutical recipes for treatment, are given below the drawings.

The seven pharmaceutical recipes added towards the end of the volume are not related to the preceding context.

***

| | |
|---|---|
| TITLE: | *Tian yi zhu you ke liu chuan ao zhi.* 天醫祝由科流傳奧旨, Profound teachings from the tradition of the specialty of invocation of the origin [of a disease with the assistance of] celestial physicians. *Zhu you shi san ke mi chuan yao jue* 祝由十三科秘傳要訣, Secretly transmitted important instructions from the 13th specialty of invocation of the origin. |
| ID: | 8954 |
| CONTENTS: | Apotropaics |
| APPEARANCE: | 2 vols. of good quality. No damage. Careful handwriting; average calligraphy. Cover: ordinary paper prepared from bamboo. No preface. |
| BINDING: | Thread |
| MEASURE: | 24.5 x 12.8 |
| TITLE PAGE: | No |
| NO. OF PAGES: | Vol. 1: 21; vol. 2: 51 |
| L.P. /CH.L: | Uneven. Writing interspersed with graphic and character charms. Lines without charms: 20/line. |
| LAYOUT: | No lines, no frames |
| AUTHOR AND YEAR OF TEXT: | |
| | Anonymous, Qing era |
| YEAR OF COPY: | We have not found characters written to comply with Qing dynasty taboos. However, the character *ning* 寧 is written in an abbreviated version. Hence for the time being we assume that this volume was written at the end of the Qing era. |

SURVEY OF CONTENTS: Both volumes are devoted to exorcism. But their contents differ. Vol. 1 has the title *Tian yi zhu you ke liu chuan ao zhi* 天醫祝由科流

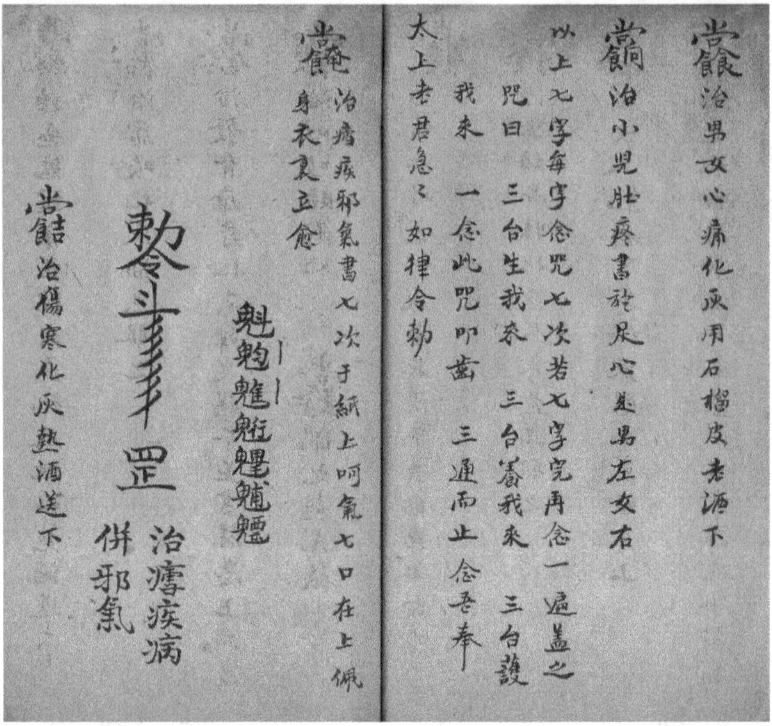

常饒治男女心痛化灰用石榴皮老酒下

常饒治小兒肚疼書於足心是男左女右
以上七字每念咒七次若七字完再念一遍盖之
咒曰　三台生我來　　三台護
我來　一念此咒叩齒　三通而止念吾奉
太上老君急之　如律令勅

常饒治瘡瘀邪氣書七次于紙上呵氣七口在上佩
常饒身衣裏立愈

魁魊魓魓魓魓

剋斗　　罡　併邪氣
　　　治瘴疾病

常饒治傷寒化灰熱酒送下

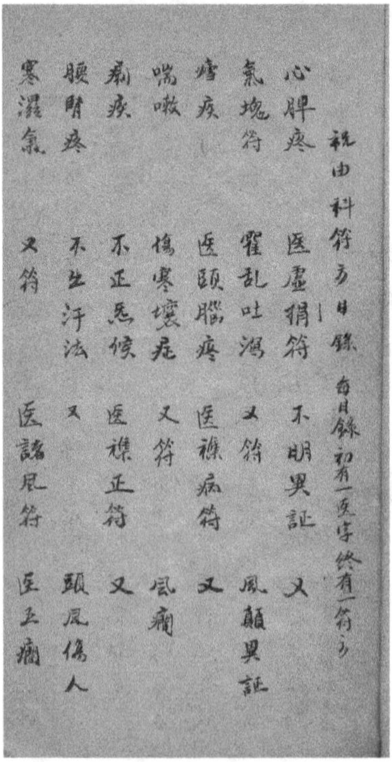

医瓦
邪牙
蚓符

嗟寧利南烏光牽捐

嗾咳那塗廣光揖

祝由科符方目錄　每日錄初一医字終有一符方
心脾寒　医盧捐符　不明異証　又
氣塊符　霍乱吐瀉　又符　風顛異証
痘疾　　医頭腦疼　医祿病符　又
喘嗽　　傷寒壞症　又符　　鼠癇
刷疾　　不正惡候　医禳正符　又
腰膝疼　不生汗法　又　　　頭屁傷人
寒濕氣　又符　　　医諸尼符　医五癇

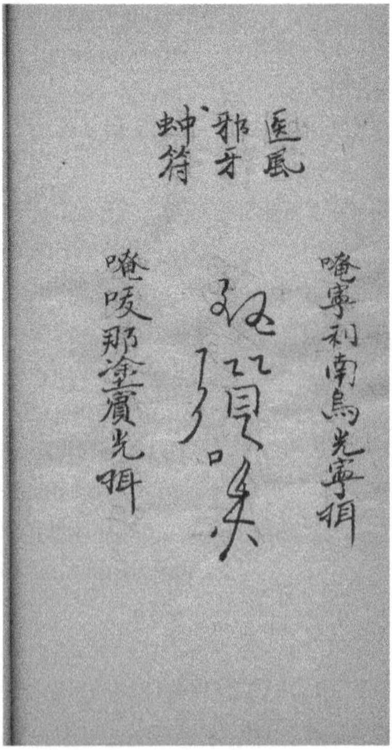

傳奧旨, "Profound teachings from the tradition of the specialty of invocation of the origin [of a disease with the assistance of] celestial physicians." It begins with a listing of former teachers of apotropaics, and a historical account, as well as major apotropaic therapy methods. The explanation of character charms is particularly detailed. Here one finds statements such as 以三字成一象，尚字為將，食字為兵，谷字為疴。以一將一兵而卻沉疴也, "one image is prepared by [joining] three characters. The character *shang* 尚 serves as an army general. The character *shi* 食 serves as soldier. The character *gu* 谷 serves as disease. With one general and one soldier it is possible to eliminate a disease". This is followed by a list of seven *jiang fu* 將符, "army general-type charms". These are characters that have the character *shang* at their top, and the character *shi* to their left. They are to be ingested together with a medication. This section is followed by another 58 charms recommended to treat a broad variety of ailments. All these charms have the character *shang* 尚 at their top. Following these "army general-type charms" graphic charms are listed to voice requests to the "celestial physicians", *tian yi* 天醫, of a total of 14 specialities, to cover a large number of ailments. This is an example of a stage in the transition from a purely apotropaic approach relying on voicing requests to the gods to a purely medical approach.

Towards the end of the first volume is a spell to stop bleeding. It may have been a contribution by the copyist himself.

The second volume has the title *Zhu you shi san ke mi chuan yao jue* 祝由十三科秘傳要訣. The contents of this volume suggest that it was copied from a text on exorcism printed during the Qing dynasty. It includes a table of contents specifying in 110 entries diseases and the charms recommended for their cure. All the charms shown in this volume are "graphic charms". Their structure shows the therapeutic indication at the top and a graphic charm below with oral spells written to the left and right. Towards the end of the volume, the structure of some of the charms is different.

The application of these charms is explained as follows: 用小薄黃紙，硃砂中書符，兩邊寫咒。各如於飲子服。如無飲子者，或茶湯，或棗湯，化符服之, "Take a thin piece of yellow paper and write the charm with cinnabar in the middle. On both sides write the oral spell, similar to the advice on application [provided in a pharmaceutical recipe]. In case no such advice on application is given, use hot tea or date decoction to ingest the dissolved [ashes of] the charm."

\*\*\*

| | |
|---|---|
| TITLE: | *She tai bian lun* 舌胎辨論, On the differentiation of tongue coatings |
| ID: | 8955 |
| CONTENTS: | Tongue diagnosis; harm caused by cold |
| APPEARANCE: | Ancient manuscript with margins somewhat damaged. Front cover stained and partially torn off. Inscription: 舌胎辨論/光□□□二月. Average calligraphy. Handwriting not very careful. No table of contents. |
| BINDING: | Thread |
| MEASURE: | 23.2 x 12.5 |
| TITLE PAGE: | No |
| NO. OF PAGES: | 28 with writing |
| L.P. /CH.L: | There are 16 pages with two tongue drawings each. Another 18 pages have text only. Below each drawing an explanatory text is given in two columns with 14 characters each. Pages without drawings mostly have 6 columns with approximately 20 characters. |
| LAYOUT: | No lines, no frames |
| AUTHOR AND YEAR OF TEXT: | |
| | Unknown |
| YEAR OF COPY: | The character 玄 is not written with a final stroke omitted to obey a Qing era taboo. The manuscript may have been written in the beginning years of the Republican era. |

SURVEY OF CONTENTS: The title of this manuscript suggests a focus on tongue coatings, but the contents are mostly concerned with harm caused by cold. The first section is *Zhi shang han zhou* 治傷寒神咒, "Divine incantation to cure harm caused by cold". This is, as the title indicates, a prayer to the gods to cure a harm caused by cold disease. It is followed by Shang han mai zheng mi lun ge 傷寒脉症秘論歌, "Secret discourse on the movement in the vessels and pathological conditions resulting from harm caused by cold, in rhymes", and She tai zheng lun 舌胎症論, "On the significance of tongue coatings as pathological signs". The latter includes a statement: 清碧李學士有云三十六舌症附之於後, "The 35 tongue conditions outlined by the scholar Li Qingbi are added at the end". Following the paragraph She tai zheng lun 舌胎症論, a survey of tongue coatings is offered. It covers 31 conditions of a "white" tongue, 25 conditions of

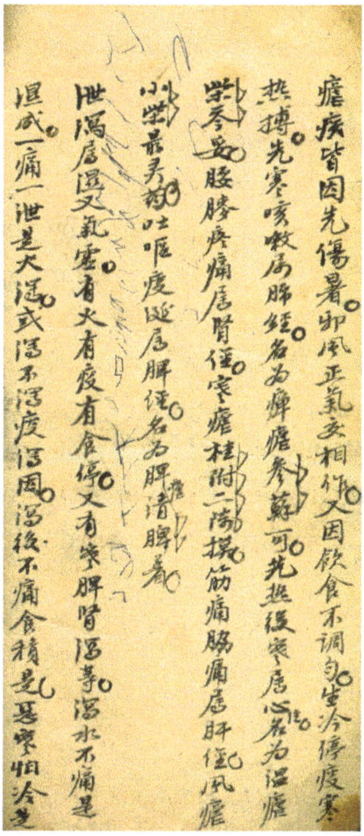

瘧疾皆因先傷暑。卻風正氣交相作。又因飲食不調勻。坐冷停痰寒熱搏。先寒咳嗽屬肺經。名為痺瘧參蘇可。先熱後寒屬心經。名為溫瘧柴苓妥。腰膝疼痛屬腎經。寒瘧桂附二陳擬。筋痛脇痛屬肝經。風瘧小柴最爲妙。吐嘔痰涎屬脾經。名爲脾清脾飲。

泄瀉屬濕又氣虛。有火有痰有食停。又有寒脾腎瀉等。瀉水不痛是濕盛。一痛一泄是火濕。或瀉不瀉痰瀉因。瀉後不痛食積是。惡寒相冷是

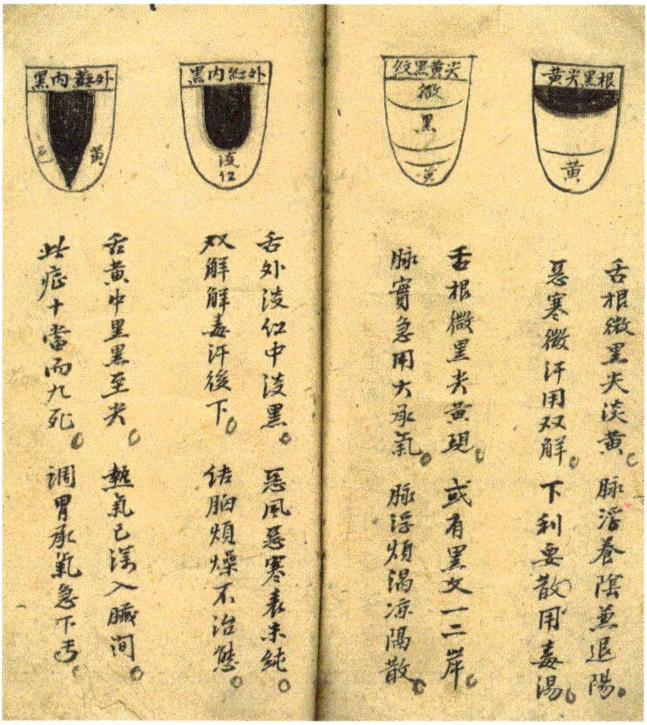



舌根微黑尖淡黃。脉滑養陰並退陽。
惡寒微汗用双解。下利要散用毒湯。
舌根微黑尖黃現。或有黑文一二岸。
脉實急用大承氣。脉浮煩渴涼隔散。

舌外淡红中淡黑。惡風惡寒表未純。
双解解毒汗後下。結胸煩燥不治然。
舌黃中黑黑至尖。熱氣已深入臟間。
此症十當而九死。調胃承氣急下之。

a "yellow" tongue, 24 conditions of a "black" tongue, 17 conditions with a grey coloring, 28 conditions with a red coloring, 12 conditions with a purple coloring, 3 with a "tainted broth", *wei jiang* 黴醬, coloring, and 3 with a blue coloring. However, the following drawings number only 36.

The section with the drawings is followed by paragraphs with the titles: Shang han qin fa shi 傷寒鈐法詩, Shang han liang gan zheng ge 傷寒兩感症歌, Shang han qin fa gui hao ge 傷寒鈐法歸號歌, Shang han qin fa kan bing an hao ge 傷寒鈐法看病安號歌, Shang han gui qin ren zi yong yao ding ju hao 傷寒歸鈐認字用藥定聚號, and Shang han yong yao miao jue 傷寒用藥妙訣. The contents of all these sections belong to non-mainstream approaches towards healing harm caused by cold that originated in the Yuan dynasty.

At the end of the manuscript two recipes are documented, as well as several couplets.


\*\*\*


| | |
|---|---|
| TITLE: | *Hua Tuo xian fang* 華佗仙方, Recipes of Hua Tuo, the immortal |
| ID: | 8956 |
| CONTENTS: | Pharmaceutical recipes |
| APPEARANCE: | A palm-size pocket book. Careful handwriting with average calligraphy. Cover made from mulberry wood paper. Stained. Inscription: 華佗仙方/楊錦雲. No preface or table of contents. |
| BINDING: | Thread |
| MEASURE: | 12,6 x 9.2 |
| TITLE PAGE: | No |
| NO. OF PAGES: | 7 |
| L.P. /CH.L: | 10 x 19 |
| LAYOUT: | Single line frames on three sides of each page enclosing a writing space of 11.0 x 8.0. |
| AUTHOR AND YEAR OF TEXT: | |
| | Wu Zhisheng 吳芝生. Date unknown. Copied by Yang Jinyun 楊錦雲. |
| YEAR OF COPY: | No hints found suggesting a time this manuscript copy may have been prepared. For the time being we presume this is an early Republican era copy. |

SURVEY OF CONTENTS: This text originates from a thin book of medical recipes prepared and published by a person intending to do something good. A line at the end of the volume reads: "A myriad copies offered reveringly by Wu Zhisheng from Xuyi in Anhui," An hui Xu yi Wu Zhisheng jing song yi wan ben

安徽盱眙吳芝生敬送壹萬本. In former times some people intending to do good to collect positive karma publicized single effective recipes free of charge so that the population benefitted from making use of them. The present volume includes 49 recipes. The therapeutic indications include the following: *wu ming zhong du* 無名腫毒, "nameless swelling with poison"; *feng huo du* 風火毒, "wind-fire poison"; *she tou ding* 蛇頭疔, "snake-head pin-illness"; *ding du e chuang* 疔毒惡瘡, "malign sore with poison associated with a pin-illness"; *zhi chuang* 痔瘡, "piles"; *lian chuang* 臁瘡, "shank sores"; *xie zhe feng zhe* 蝎蜇蜂蜇, "scorpion-sting; bee sting"; *kou chuang* 口瘡, "oral lesions"; *huang shui chuang* 黃水瘡, "lesions with yellow water"; *huo shao shui tang* 火燒水燙, "burns"; *die da sun shang* 跌打損傷, "injuries from falls and blows"; *ye shi fan wei* 噎食反胃, "burping and stomach reflux"; *fu ren lao xue* 婦人癆血, "consumption with bleeding of women"; *zhen zha rou nei* 針扎肉內, "needle stuck in the flesh"; and other commonly encountered health problems. The recipes recommended are mostly single substance recipes, and the substances used are mostly those easily obtained in one's environment. There are also some commonly prepared medications to be bought in a pharmacy.

***

| | |
|---|---|
| TITLE: | *Shen ying jing* 神應經, Classic on divine responses |
| ID: | 8957 |
| CONTENTS: | Acupuncture |
| APPEARANCE: | Ancient manuscript. Cover prepared from locally produced paper. No title. Average calligraphy. |
| BINDING: | Paper spills, with later cover pasted around two metal wire threads running along the spine. |
| MEASURE: | 17.9 x 13.4 |
| TITLE PAGE: | No |
| NO. OF PAGES: | 48 |
| L.P. /CH.L: | 9 x 21 |
| LAYOUT: | No lines, no frames |
| AUTHOR AND YEAR OF TEXT: | |
| | Chen Hui 陳會 (1425), Ming era. Amended and edited by Liu Jin 劉瑾. |
| YEAR OF COPY: | No Qing dynasty taboos observed. Republican era. |

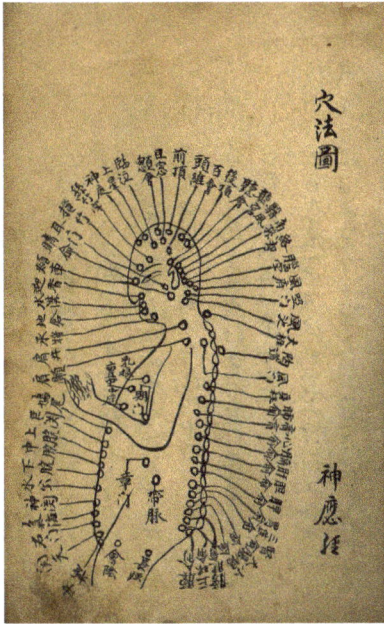

SURVEY OF CONTENTS: This volume is on acupuncture. It begins with a head-ing Shou jue 手訣, "manual gestures", followed by the following five sections: San guan 三關, "Three passes", Liu fu 六府, "Six palaces", Ti tou 剃頭, "Shaving the head", Hu yang 護養, "Saving and nourishing", and Ren jin fa ge 認筋法歌, "Method to recognize the [location] patterns of sinews, in rhymes". All these are *tui na* 推拿 push-and-pull massage techniques. They are unrelated to the remaining contents of this volume.

This initial section is followed by a table of contents and the naming of a title *Zhen jiu da cheng* 鍼灸大成. However, a close inspection shows that this is not a faithful copy of the text *Zhen jiu da cheng* 鍼灸大成 compiled by Yang Jizhou 楊繼洲 and edited by Jin Xian 靳賢. Rather, this is a partial copy of the *Shen ying jing* 神應經 written by the Ming author Chen Hui 陳會 and pub-lished in 1425, as amended by Liu Jin 劉瑾.

The table of contents of the present volume begins with the paragraph Xue fa tu 穴法圖, "Drawings of the [location] patterns of [insertion] holes". This is followed by drawings showing the course of the 12 conduits by pointing out in detail the locations of their insertion holes and offering advice on needling techniques. This is followed by a catalogue of disease names and advice on which needle insertion holes are to be chosen for their acupuncture treatment. In general, the contents of the present volume appear somewhat abridged in comparison with the original text of the *Shen ying jing* 神應經.

\*\*\*

| | |
|---|---|
| TITLE: | *Shang lun pian* 尚論篇, Treasured discourse |
| ID: | 8958 |
| CONTENTS: | Harm caused by cold |
| APPEARANCE: | Fine manscript in four volumes in a cardboard case covered by blue linen fabric. The paper appears aged but the volumes are in good condition nevertheless. Excellent calligraphy. |
| BINDING: | Thread |
| MEASURE: | 17,7 x 13,0 |
| TITLE PAGE: | Cover and first page without book title. |
| NO. OF PAGES: | 240: Vol. 1: 54; vol. 2: 66; vol. 3: 69; vol. 4: 51. |
| L.P. /CH.L: | 10 x 20 |
| LAYOUT: | No lines, no frames |

AUTHOR AND YEAR OF TEXT:

Qing dynasty, Yu Chang 喻昌; name of copyist unknown.

YEAR OF COPY:     Throughout this manuscript the character 玄 *xuan* is either changed in its appreance or written with the final stroke omitted to observe a Qing dynasty taboo. Hence the text appears to have been written towards the end of the Qing dynasty.

SURVEY OF CONTENTS: This is a copy of the famous Ming dynasty physician Yu Chang's 喻昌, *zi*: Jiayan 嘉言, work *Shang lun pian* 尚論篇 in 4 *juan*. The complete title of this book reads *Shang lun Zhang Zhong jing shang han lun chong pian san bai jiu shi qi fa* 尚論張仲景傷寒論重編三百九十七法. It is a discourse on the therapeutic patterns and implicit meaning of Zhang Zhongjing's 張仲景 *Shang han lun* 傷寒論. This book was published and widely spread in printed editions during the Qing era. Apparently, individual readers also prepared fine manuscript copies, such as this one. Maybe the copyist had a special liking for this book and hence did not hesitate to prepare a copy of the full text. Still, the text copied here does not entirely agree with the original; it has some omissions.

***

TITLE:             (*Min jian yao fang* 民間藥方, Folk pharmaceutical recipes)
ID:                8959
CONTENTS:          Pharmaceutical recipes
APPEARANCE:        Ancient manuscript. Cover and title page torn off. Margins and edges severely damaged. Ancient handwriting of different levels; at times fine, at times crude and careless.
BINDING:           Thread
MEASURE:           23.0 x 12.2
TITLE PAGE:        No
NO. OF PAGES:      62
L.P. /CH.L:        Number of lines uneven, often from 5 to 7. Characters per line similarly uneven. Often up to 25.
LAYOUT:            No lines; no frames
AUTHOR AND YEAR OF TEXT:

Qing dynasty, unknown

YEAR OF COPY:　　The nature and contents of these recipes suggest that this volume was written towards the end of the Qing dynasty or in the early years of the Republic.

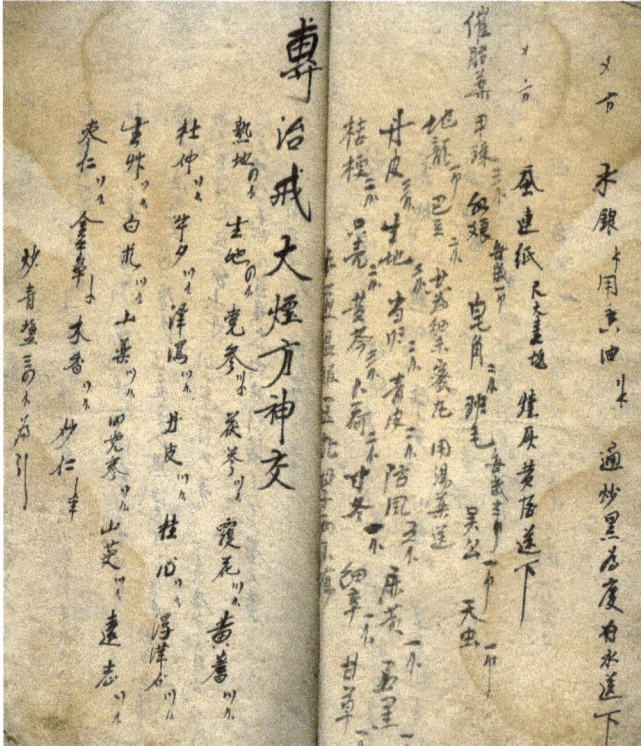

SURVEY OF CONTENTS: This is a record of approximately 270 miscellaneous pharmaceutical recipes. Apparently, the recipes were casually written down and hence there is no structure discernible in their listing. In general, the contents of this volume are rather chaotic. The nature of the recipes documented is quite heterogenous. Some are set prescriptions, others are prescriptions with many ingredients, and still others are folk recipes based on only a few substances or with only one single ingredient. Prescriptions to stop the consumption of "foreign tobacco", *yang yan* 洋菸, suggest that this manuscript was written towards the end of the Qing dynasty.

Also, among the recipes one finds records unrelated to pharmaceutical therapy, including charms and incantations and others listed under the following headings: 嫁神方位、糞神日、嫁娶天相不和、婦人上頭避忌、人死時辰、四季天坑方位、天干、八卦.

*\*\**

| | |
|---|---|
| TITLE: | *Zhang tian shi tui bing fang* 張天師退病方, Heavenly teacher Zhang's recipes to turn away disease |
| ID: | 8960 |
| CONTENTS: | Exorcism |
| APPEARANCE: | Ancient manuscript. Cover stained. Inscription upper left: 張天師退病方/民國丙寅年訂. Average calligraphy. 60 handdrawn illustrations of demon images. |
| BINDING: | Thread |
| MEASURE: | 18.2 x 12.5 |
| TITLE PAGE: | No |
| NO. OF PAGES: | 29 |
| L.P. /CH.L: | 4 – 7 x up to 18 |
| LAYOUT: | No lines, no frames |
| AUTHOR AND YEAR OF TEXT: | |
| | Unknown |
| YEAR OF COPY: | The volume has a date on its cover: 丙寅年訂. That is 1926. |

SURVEY OF CONTENTS: This manuscript volume focusses on the causes of and reactions to ailments caused demon spirits. Such contents are a specialty of folk exorcistic healers. The current volume is of the same type as an earlier volume in this collection, ID 8554, i.e., *Fa bing shu* 法病書. A comparison shows that they are identical in many respects. For example, both volumes calculate, on the basis of the day on which a disease emerged, which demon in a circular period of 60 days may have caused this disease. The days are counted according to the 60 days cycle named with the combination of heavenly stems and earth branches. Each day gives the symptoms of the disease, the position of the responsible demon in the patient's house, and the method how to expel the demon. Hence both volumes combine one illustration of a demon in question with one explanatory text. The texts and the illustrations are basically the same in both volumes. Only the details in the drawings, such as the coloring and the gestures of the demons, may differ. This suggests that the current volume and volume 8554 have one identical source.

However, if compared with the *Fa bing shu* 法病書, the current volume lists three demons less, and has omitted drawings and texts related to the two days *bing zi* 丙子 and *ding chou* 丁丑. Also, at its very end it lacks the final *wang ba* 王霸, "despot king", demon. The quality of the illustrations is inferior to that of

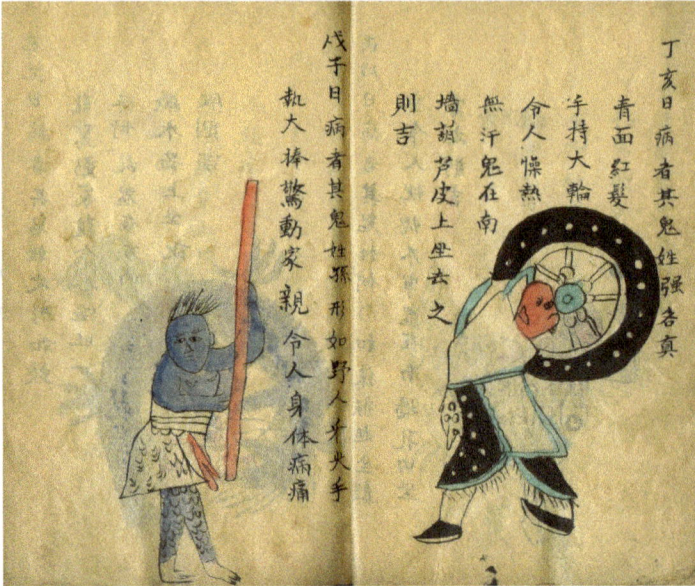

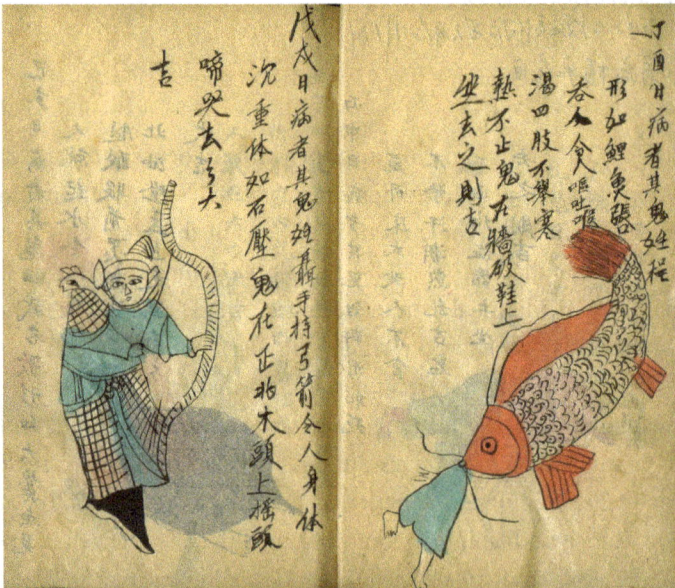

the *Fa bing shu* 法病書. The colors are not as variegated and brilliant as in *Fa bing shu* 法病書.

A comparison of two texts may show the degree of differences between the two volumes. For example, the *Fa bing shu* 法病書 states:

丁未日，病者其鬼姓耿，名田，形如美貌女子，時常好笑。令人頭疼身重，口苦無味。鬼在病人衣服上坐，去之大吉

"*Ding wei* day: The name of the demon responsible for the disease is Geng, his personal name is Tian. His appearance is that of a good looking female. It often laughs. It causes humans to have headache and a heavy body. The mouth suffers from being unable to distinguish flavors. The demon sits on the patient's garments. To remove them is very auspicious."

*The Zhang tian shi tui bing fa* 張天師退病法 has:

丁未日，病者其鬼姓耿，名冉，形如美女，時常似笑。令人沉重，口苦無味。鬼在病人花衣上坐，去衣即好

"*Ding wei* day: The name of the demon responsible for the disease is Geng, his personal name is Rang. His appearance is that of a beautiful female. It often appears as if laughing. It causes humans to feel a severe heaviness. The mouth suffers from being unable to distinguish flavors. The demon sits on the patient's adorned garments. After the garments have been removed [the patient] will feel fine again."

The present volume appears to have been prepared more recently than the *Fa bing shu* 法病書. Both deserve a more careful comparion.

# Index of Authors, Copyists and Owners

# INDEX OF SUBJECTS

# Index of Titles

www.ingramcontent.com/pod-product-compliance
Lightning Source LLC
Chambersburg PA
CBHW050659190326
41458CB00008B/2618